# ATHEROSCLEROSIS
# &
# CORONARY ARTERY DISEASES

## Everything About Patient's Instruction
## After cardiac Procedures

BY DR MOHAMMED MAJEED

# Terms and Conditions
## <u>LEGAL NOTICE</u>

# Table of Contents

# INDEX

# ATHEROSCLEROSIS

## What is Atherosclerosis

Atherosclerosis is narrowing and hardening of the arteries. Arteries are blood vessels that carry blood from the heart to all parts of the body. This blood contains oxygen. Arteries can become narrow or clogged with a buildup of fat, cholesterol, calcium, and other substances (*plaque*). Plaque decreases the amount of blood that can flow through the artery.

Atherosclerosis can affect any artery in the body, including:

- Heart arteries (*coronary artery disease*). This may cause a heart attack.
- Brain arteries. This may cause a stroke (*cerebrovascular accident*).
- Leg, arm, and pelvis arteries (*peripheral artery disease*). This may cause pain and numbness.
- Kidney arteries. This may cause kidney (*renal*) failure.

Treatment may slow the disease and prevent further damage to the heart, brain, peripheral arteries, and kidneys.

## What are the causes?

Atherosclerosis develops slowly over many years. The inner layers of your arteries become damaged and allow the gradual buildup of plaque. The exact cause of atherosclerosis is not fully understood. Symptoms of atherosclerosis do not occur until the artery becomes narrow or blocked.

# What increases the risk?

The following factors may make you more likely to develop this condition:

- High blood pressure.
- High cholesterol.
- Being middle-aged or older.
- Having a family history of atherosclerosis.
- Having high blood fats (*triglycerides*).
- Diabetes.
- Being overweight.
- Smoking tobacco.
- Not exercising enough (*sedentary lifestyle*).
- Having a substance in the blood called C-reactive protein (CRP). This is a sign of increased levels of inflammation in the body.
- Sleep apnea.
- Being stressed.
- Drinking too much alcohol.
- This condition may not cause any symptoms. If you have symptoms, they are caused by damage to an area of your body that is not getting enough blood.
- Coronary artery disease may cause chest pain and shortness of breath.
- Decreased blood supply to your brain may cause a stroke. Signs of a stroke may include sudden:
- Weakness on one side of the body.
- Confusion.
- Changes in vision.
- Inability to speak or understand speech.
- Loss of balance, coordination, or the ability to walk.
- Severe headache.
- Loss of consciousness.

- Peripheral arterial disease may cause pain and numbness, often in the legs and hips.
- Renal failure may cause fatigue, nausea, swelling, and itchy skin.

## How is this diagnosed?

This condition is diagnosed based on your medical history and a physical exam. During the exam:

- Your health care provider will:
- Check your pulse in different places.
- Listen for a "whooshing" sound over your arteries (*bruit*).
- You may have tests, such as:
- Blood tests to check your levels of cholesterol, triglycerides, and CRP.
- Electrocardiogram (ECG) to check for heart damage.
- Chest X-ray to see if you have an enlarged heart, which is a sign of heart failure.
- Stress test to see how your heart reacts to exercise.
- Echocardiogram to get images of the inside of your heart.
- Ankle-brachial index to compare blood pressure in your arms to blood pressure in your ankles.
- Ultrasound of your peripheral arteries to check blood flow.
- CT scan to check for damage to your heart or brain.
- X-rays of blood vessels after dye has been injected (*angiogram*) to check blood flow.

# Heart Attack

The heart is a muscle that needs oxygen to survive. A heart attack is a condition that occurs when your heart does not get enough oxygen. When this happens, the heart muscle begins to die. This can cause permanent damage if not treated right away. A heart attack is a medical emergency.

This condition may be called a myocardial infarction, or MI. It is also known as acute coronary syndrome (ACS). ACS is a term used to describe a group of conditions that affect blood flow to the heart.

## What are the causes?

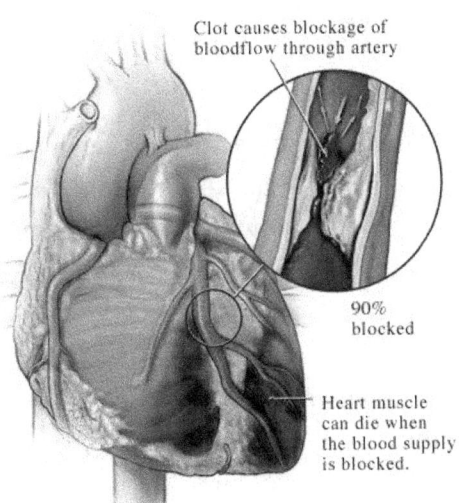

Clot causes blockage of bloodflow through artery

90% blocked

Heart muscle can die when the blood supply is blocked.

This condition may be caused by:

- Atherosclerosis. This occurs when a fatty substance called plaque builds up in the arteries and blocks or reduces blood supply to the heart.

- A blood clot. A blood clot can develop suddenly when plaque breaks up within an artery and blocks blood flow to the heart.
- Low blood pressure.
- An abnormal heartbeat (*arrhythmia*).
- Conditions that cause a decrease of oxygen to the heart, such as anemia or respiratory failure.
- A spasm, or severe tightening, of a blood vessel that cuts off blood flow to the heart.
- Tearing of a coronary artery (spontaneous coronary artery dissection).
- High blood pressure.

## What increases the risk?

The following factors may make you more likely to develop this condition:

- Aging. The older you are, the higher your risk.
- Having a personal or family history of chest pain, heart attack, stroke, or narrowing of the arteries in the legs, arms, head, or stomach (*peripheral artery disease*).
- Being male.
- Smoking.
- Not getting regular exercise.
- Being overweight or obese.
- Having high blood pressure.
- Having high cholesterol (*hypercholesterolemia*).
- Having diabetes.
- Drinking too much alcohol.
- Using illegal drugs, such as cocaine or methamphetamine.

# What are the signs or symptoms?

Symptoms of this condition may vary, depending on factors like gender and age. Symptoms may include:

- Chest pain. It may feel like:
  - Crushing or squeezing.
  - Tightness, pressure, fullness, or heaviness.
- Pain in the arm, neck, jaw, back, or upper body.
- Shortness of breath.
- Heartburn or upset stomach.
- Nausea.
- Sudden cold sweats.
- Feeling tired.
- Sudden light-headedness.

# How is this diagnosed?

This condition may be diagnosed through tests, such as:

- Electrocardiogram (ECG) to measure the electrical activity of your heart.
- Blood tests to check for cardiac markers. These chemicals are released by a damaged heart muscle.
- A test to evaluate blood flow and heart function (*coronary angiogram*).
- CT scan to see the heart more clearly.
- A test to evaluate the pumping action of the heart (*echocardiogram*).

# How is this treated?

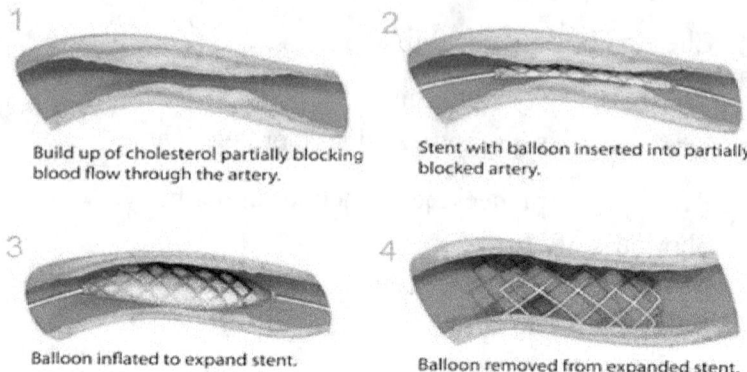

Stent with Balloon Angioplasty

1
Build up of cholesterol partially blocking blood flow through the artery.

2
Stent with balloon inserted into partially blocked artery.

3
Balloon inflated to expand stent.

4
Balloon removed from expanded stent.

A heart attack must be treated as soon as possible. Treatment may include:

- Medicines to:
  - ➤ Break up or dissolve blood clots (*fibrinolytic therapy*).
  - ➤ Thin blood and help prevent blood clots.
  - ➤ Treat blood pressure.
  - ➤ Improve blood flow to the heart.
  - ➤ Reduce pain.
  - ➤ Reduce cholesterol.
- Angioplasty and stent placement. These are procedures to widen a blocked artery and keep it open.
- Coronary artery bypass graft, CABG, or open heart surgery. This enables blood to flow to the heart by going around the blocked part of the artery.
- Oxygen therapy if needed.
- Cardiac rehabilitation. This improves your health and well-being through exercise, education, and counseling.

# Follow these instructions at home:

## Medicines

- Take over-the-counter and prescription medicines only as told by your health care provider.
- **Do not** take the following medicines unless your health care provider says it is okay to take them:
  - ➢ NSAIDs, such as ibuprofen.
  - ➢ Supplements that contain vitamin A, vitamin E, or both.
  - ➢ Hormone replacement therapy that contains estrogen with or without progestin.

## Lifestyle

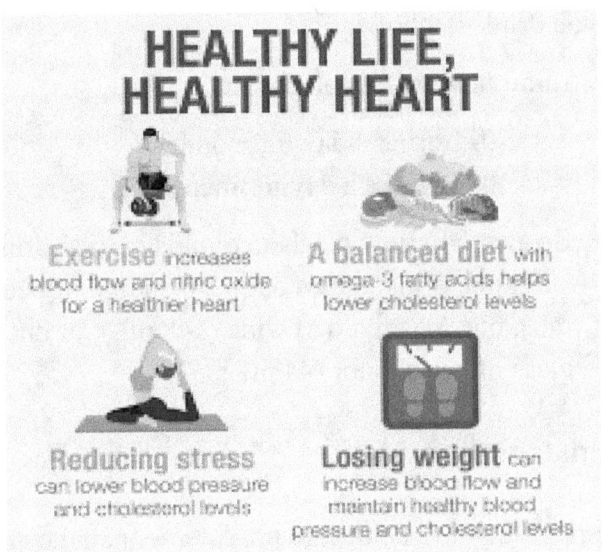

- **Do not** use any products that contain nicotine or tobacco, such as cigarettes, e-cigarettes, and chewing tobacco. If you need help quitting, ask your health care provider.
- Avoid secondhand smoke.

- Exercise regularly. Ask your health care provider about participating in a cardiac rehabilitation program that helps you start exercising safely after a heart attack.
- Eat a heart-healthy diet. Your health care provider will tell you what foods to eat.
- Maintain a healthy weight.
- Learn ways to manage stress.
- **Do not** use illegal drugs.

### Alcohol use

- **Do not** drink alcohol if:
  - ➤ Your health care provider tells you not to drink.
  - ➤ You are pregnant, may be pregnant, or are planning to become pregnant.
- If you drink alcohol:
  - ➤ Limit how much you use to:
    - o 0–1 drink a day for women.
    - o 0–2 drinks a day for men.
  - ➤ Be aware of how much alcohol is in your drink. In the U.S., one drink equals one 12 oz bottle of beer (355 mL), one 5 oz glass of wine (148 mL), or one 1½ oz glass of hard liquor (44 mL).

## General instructions

- Work with your health care provider to manage any other conditions you have, such as high blood pressure or diabetes. These conditions affect your heart.
- Get screened for depression, and seek treatment if needed.
- Keep your vaccinations up to date. Get the flu vaccine every year.

- Keep all follow-up visits as told by your health care provider. This is important.

## Contact a health care provider if:

- You feel overwhelmed or sad.
- You have trouble doing your daily activities.

## Get help right away if:

- You have sudden, unexplained discomfort in your chest, arms, back, neck, jaw, or upper body.
- You have shortness of breath.
- You suddenly start to sweat or your skin gets clammy.
- You feel nauseous or you vomit.
- You have unexplained tiredness or weakness.
- You suddenly feel light-headed or dizzy.
- You notice your heart starts to beat fast or feels like it is skipping beats.
- You have blood pressure that is higher than 180/120.

**These symptoms may represent a serious problem that is an emergency. Do not wait to see if the symptoms will go away. Get medical help right away. Call your local emergency services (911 in the U.S.). Do not drive yourself to the hospital.**

## Summary

- A heart attack, also called myocardial infarction, is a condition that occurs when your heart does not get enough oxygen. This is caused by anything that blocks or reduces blood flow to the heart.

- Treatment is a combination of medicines and surgeries, if needed, to open the blocked arteries and restore blood flow to the heart.
- A heart attack is an emergency. Get help right away if you have sudden discomfort in your chest, arms, back, neck, jaw, or upper body. Seek help if you feel nauseous, you vomit, or you feel light-headed or dizzy.

## How is this treated?

- Treatment starts with lifestyle changes, which may include:
- Changing your diet.
- Losing weight.
- Reducing stress.
- Exercising and being physically active more regularly.
- Not smoking.
- You may also need medicine to:

  ➢ Lower triglycerides and cholesterol.
  ➢ Control blood pressure.
  ➢ Prevent blood clots.
  ➢ Lower inflammation in your body.
  ➢ Control your blood sugar.

- Sometimes, surgery is needed to:

  ➢ Remove plaque from an artery (*endarterectomy*).
  ➢ Open or widen a narrowed heart artery (*angioplasty*).
  ➢ Create a new path for your blood with one of these procedures:

    ○ Heart (*coronary*) artery bypass graft surgery.
    ○ Peripheral artery bypass graft surgery.

# Follow these instructions at home:

## Eating and drinking

- Eat a heart-healthy diet. Talk with your health care provider or a diet and nutrition specialist (*dietitian*) if you need help. A heart-healthy diet involves:
  - ➢ Limiting unhealthy fats and increasing healthy fats. Some examples of healthy fats are olive oil and canola oil.
  - ➢ Eating plant-based foods, such as fruits, vegetables, nuts, whole grains, and legumes (such as peas and lentils).
- Limit alcohol intake to no more than 1 drink a day for nonpregnant women and 2 drinks a day for men. One drink equals 12 oz of beer, 5 oz of wine, or 1½ oz of hard liquor.

## Lifestyle

- Follow an exercise program as told by your health care provider.
- Maintain a healthy weight. Lose weight if your health care provider says that you need to do that.
- Rest when you are tired.
- Learn to manage your stress.
- **Do not** use any products that contain nicotine or tobacco, such as cigarettes and e- cigarettes. If you need help quitting, ask your health care provider.
- **Do not** abuse drugs.

# General instructions

- Take over-the-counter and prescription medicines only as told by your health care provider.

- Manage other health conditions as told by your health care provider.
- Keep all follow-up visits as told by your health care provider. This is important.

## Contact a health care provider if:

- You have chest pain or discomfort. This includes squeezing chest pain that may feel like indigestion (*angina*).
- You have shortness of breath.
- You have an irregular heartbeat.
- You have unexplained fatigue.
- You have unexplained pain or numbness in an arm, leg, or hip.
- You have nausea, swelling of your hands or feet, and itchy skin.

## Get help right away if:

- You have any symptoms of a heart attack, such as:
  - ➢ Chest pain.
  - ➢ Shortness of breath.
  - ➢ Pain in your neck, jaw, arms, back, or stomach.
  - ➢ Cold sweat.
  - ➢ Nausea.
  - ➢ Light-headedness.
- You have any symptoms of a stroke. **"BE FAST"** is an easy way to remember the main warning signs of a stroke:
  - ➢ **B - Balance.** Signs are dizziness, sudden trouble walking, or loss of balance.
  - ➢ **E - Eyes.** Signs are trouble seeing or a sudden change in vision.

- ➢ **F - Face.** Signs are sudden weakness or numbness of the face, or the face or eyelid drooping on one side.
- ➢ **A - Arms.** Signs are weakness or numbness in an arm. This happens suddenly and usually on one side of the body.
- ➢ **S - Speech.** Signs are sudden trouble speaking, slurred speech, or trouble understanding what people say.
- ➢ **T - Time.** Time to call emergency services. Write down what time symptoms started.

- You have other signs of a stroke, such as:

  - ➢ A sudden, severe headache with no known cause.
  - ➢ Nausea or vomiting.

# Coronary Artery Disease (Male)

Coronary artery disease (CAD) is a condition in which the arteries that lead to the heart (*coronary arteries*) become narrow or blocked. The narrowing or blockage can lead to decreased blood flow to the heart. Prolonged reduced blood flow can cause a heart attack (*myocardial infarction* or *MI*). This condition may also be called coronary heart disease.

Because CAD is the leading cause of death in men, it is important to understand what causes this condition and how it is treated.

## What are the causes?

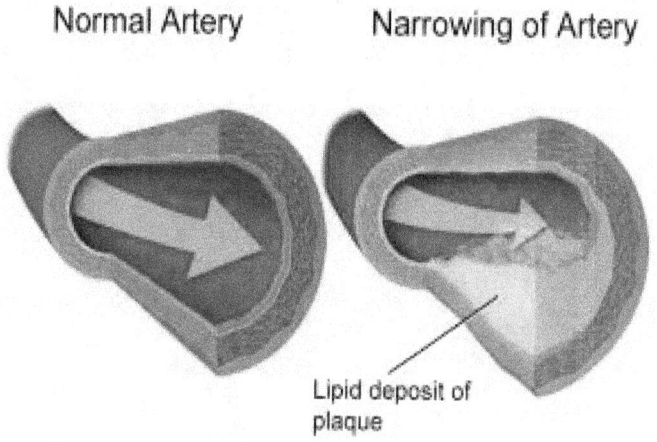

Normal Artery      Narrowing of Artery

Lipid deposit of plaque

**Coronary Artery Disease**

CAD is most often caused by atherosclerosis. This is the buildup of fat and cholesterol (*plaque*) on the inside of the arteries. Over time, the plaque may narrow or block the artery, reducing blood flow to the heart. Plaque can also become weak and break off within a coronary artery and cause a sudden blockage. Other less common causes of CAD include:

- A blood clot or a piece of a blood clot or other substance that blocks the flow of blood in a coronary artery (*embolism*).
- A tearing of the artery (spontaneous coronary artery dissection).
- An enlargement of an artery (*aneurysm*).
- Inflammation (*vasculitis*) in the artery wall.

## What increases the risk?

The following factors may make you more likely to develop this condition:

- Age. Men over age 45 are at a greater risk of CAD.
- Family history of CAD.
- Gender. Men often develop CAD earlier in life than women.
- High blood pressure (*hypertension*).
- Diabetes.
- High cholesterol levels.
- Tobacco use.
- Excessive alcohol use.
- Lack of exercise.
- A diet high in saturated and *trans* fats, such as fried food and processed meat.

Other possible risk factors include:

- High stress levels.
- Depression.
- Obesity.
- Sleep apnea.

# What are the signs or symptoms?

Many people do not have any symptoms during the early stages of CAD. As the condition progresses, symptoms may include:

- Chest pain (*angina*). The pain can:
  - Feel like crushing or squeezing, or like a tightness, pressure, fullness, or heaviness in the chest.
  - Last more than a few minutes or can stop and recur. The pain tends to get worse with exercise or stress and to fade with rest.

- Pain in the arms, neck, jaw, ear, or back.
- Unexplained heartburn or indigestion.
- Shortness of breath.
- Nausea or vomiting.
- Sudden light-headedness.
- Sudden cold sweats.
- Fluttering or fast heartbeat (*palpitations*).

# How is this diagnosed?

This condition is diagnosed based on:

- Your family and medical history.
- A physical exam.
- Tests, including:
  - A test to check the electrical signals in your heart (*electrocardiogram*).
  - Exercise stress test. This looks for signs of blockage when the heart is stressed with exercise, such as running on a treadmill.
  - Pharmacologic stress test. This test looks for signs of blockage when the heart is being stressed with a medicine.

- ➤ Blood tests.
- ➤ Coronary angiogram. This is a procedure to look at the coronary arteries to see if there is any blockage. During this test, a dye is injected into your arteries so they appear on an X-ray.
- ➤ Coronary artery CT scan. This CT scan helps detect calcium deposits in your coronary arteries. Calcium deposits are an indicator of CAD.
- ➤ A test that uses sound waves to take a picture of your heart (*echocardiogram*).
- ➤ Chest X-ray.

## How is this treated?

This condition may be treated by:

- Healthy lifestyle changes to reduce risk factors.
- Medicines such as:
  - ➤ Antiplatelet medicines and blood-thinning medicines, such as aspirin. These help to prevent blood clots.
  - ➤ Nitroglycerin.
  - ➤ Blood pressure medicines.
  - ➤ Cholesterol-lowering medicine.
- Coronary angioplasty and stenting. During this procedure, a thin, flexible tube is inserted through a blood vessel and into a blocked artery. A balloon or similar device on the end of the tube is inflated to open up the artery. In some cases, a small, mesh tube (*stent*) is inserted into the artery to keep it open.
- Coronary artery bypass surgery. During this surgery, veins or arteries from other parts of the body are used to create a bypass around the blockage and allow blood to reach your heart.

# Follow these instructions at home:

## Medicines

- Take over-the-counter and prescription medicines only as told by your health care provider.
- **Do not** take the following medicines unless your health care provider approves:
  - ➢ NSAIDs, such as ibuprofen, naproxen, or celecoxib.
  - ➢ Vitamin supplements that contain vitamin A, vitamin E, or both.

## Lifestyle

- Follow an exercise program approved by your health care provider. Aim for 150 minutes of moderate exercise or 75 minutes of vigorous exercise each week.
- Maintain a healthy weight or lose weight as approved by your health care provider.
- Learn to manage stress or try to limit your stress. Ask your health care provider for suggestions if you need help.
- Get screened for depression and seek treatment, if needed.
- **Do not** use any products that contain nicotine or tobacco, such as cigarettes, e-cigarettes, and chewing tobacco. If you need help quitting, ask your health care provider.
- **Do not** use illegal drugs.

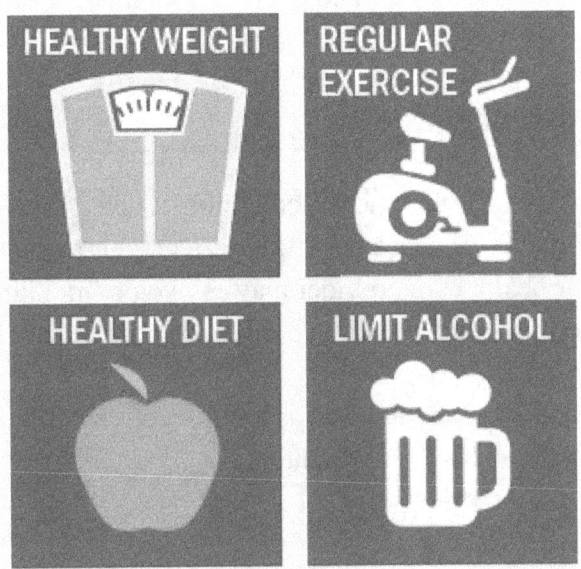

- Follow a heart-healthy diet. A dietitian can help educate you about healthy food options and changes. In general, eat plenty of fruits and vegetables, lean meats, and whole grains.
- Avoid foods high in:
  - Sugar.
  - Salt (*sodium*).
  - Saturated fat, such as processed or fatty meat.
  - *Trans* fat, such as fried foods.
- Use healthy cooking methods such as roasting, grilling, broiling, baking, poaching, steaming, or stir-frying.
- **Do not** drink alcohol if your health care provider tells you not to drink.
- If you drink alcohol:
  - Limit how much you have to 0–2 drinks per day.

➤ Be aware of how much alcohol is in your drink. In the U.S., one drink equals one 12 oz bottle of beer (355 mL), one 5 oz glass of wine (148 mL), or one 1½ oz glass of hard liquor (44 mL).

## General instructions

- Manage any other health conditions, such as hypertension and diabetes. These conditions affect your heart.
- Your health care provider may ask you to monitor your blood pressure. Ideally, your blood pressure should be below 130/80.
- Keep all follow-up visits as told by your health care provider. This is important.

## Get help right away if:

- You have pain in your chest, neck, ear, arm, jaw, stomach, or back that:
  - ➤ Lasts more than a few minutes.
  - ➤ Is recurring.
  - ➤ Is not relieved by taking medicine under your tongue (*sublingual nitroglycerin*).
- You have profuse sweating without cause.
- You have unexplained:
  - ➤ Heartburn or indigestion.
  - ➤ Shortness of breath or difficulty breathing.
  - ➤ Fluttering or fast heartbeat (*palpitations*).
  - ➤ Nausea or vomiting.
  - ➤ Fatigue.
  - ➤ Feelings of nervousness or anxiety.
  - ➤ Weakness.
  - ➤ Diarrhea.

- You have sudden light-headedness or dizziness.
- You faint.
- You feel like hurting yourself or think about taking your own life.

**These symptoms may represent a serious problem that is an emergency. Do not wait to see if the symptoms will go away. Get medical help right away. Call your local emergency services (911 in the U.S.). Do not drive yourself to the hospital.**

## Summary

- Coronary artery disease (CAD) is a condition in which the arteries that lead to the heart (*coronary arteries*) become narrow or blocked. The narrowing or blockage can lead to a heart attack.
- Many people do not have any symptoms during the early stages of CAD.
- CAD can be treated with lifestyle changes, medicines, surgery, or a combination of these treatments.

This information is not intended to replace advice given to you by your health care provider. Make sure you discuss any questions you have with your health care provider.

# Acute Coronary Syndrome

Acute coronary syndrome (ACS) is a serious problem in which there is suddenly not enough blood and oxygen reaching the heart. ACS can result in chest pain or a heart attack.

This condition is a medical emergency. If you have any symptoms of this condition, get help right away.

## What are the causes?

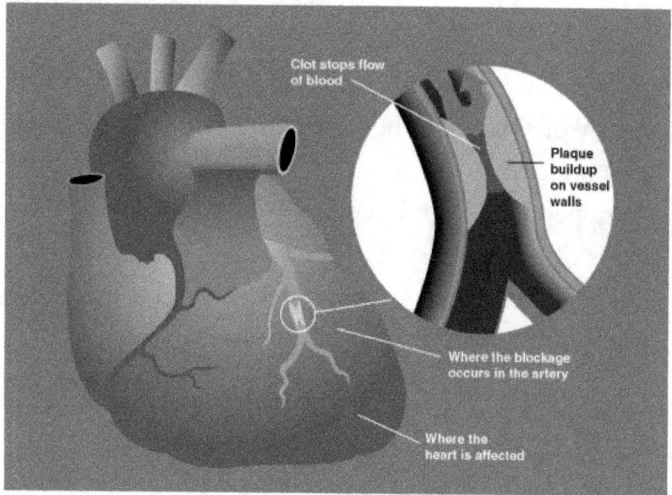

This condition may be caused by:

- A buildup of fat and cholesterol inside the arteries (*atherosclerosis*). This is the most common cause. The buildup (*plaque*) can cause blood vessels in the heart (*coronary arteries*) to become narrow or blocked, which reduces blood flow to the heart. Plaque can also break off and lead to a clot, which can block an artery and cause a heart attack or stroke.

- Sudden tightening of the muscles around the coronary arteries (*coronary spasm*).
- Tearing of a coronary artery (*spontaneous coronary artery dissection*).
- Very low blood pressure (*hypotension*).
- An abnormal heartbeat (*arrhythmia*).
- Other medical conditions that cause a decrease of oxygen to the heart, such as anemia or respiratory failure.
- Using cocaine or methamphetamine.

## What increases the risk?

The following factors may make you more likely to develop this condition:

- Age. The risk for ACS increases as you get older.
- History of chest pain, heart attack, peripheral artery disease, or stroke.
- Having taken chemotherapy or immune-suppressing medicines.
- Being male.
- Family history of chest pain, heart disease, or stroke.
- Smoking.
- Not exercising enough.
- Being overweight.
- High cholesterol.
- High blood pressure (*hypertension*).
- Diabetes.
- Excessive alcohol use.

## What are the signs or symptoms?

Common symptoms of this condition include:

- Chest pain. The pain may last a long time, or it may stop and come back (*recur*). It may feel like:
  - ➤ Crushing or squeezing.
  - ➤ Tightness, pressure, fullness, or heaviness.
- Arm, neck, jaw, or back pain.
- Heartburn or indigestion.
- Shortness of breath.
- Nausea.
- Sudden cold sweats.
- Light-headedness.
- Dizziness or passing out.
- Tiredness (*fatigue*).

Sometimes there are no symptoms.

## How is this diagnosed?

This condition may be diagnosed based on:

- Your medical history and symptoms.
- Imaging tests, such as:
  - ➤ An electrocardiogram (ECG). This measures the heart's electrical activity.
  - ➤ X-rays.
  - ➤ CT scan.
  - ➤ A coronary angiogram. For this test, dye is injected into the heart arteries and then X-rays are taken.
  - ➤ Myocardial perfusion imaging. This test shows how well blood flows through your heart muscle.
- Blood tests. These may be repeated at certain time intervals.

- Exercise stress testing.
- Echocardiogram. This is a test that uses sound waves to produce detailed images of the heart.

## How is this treated?

Treatment for this condition may include:

- Oxygen therapy.
- Medicines, such as:
  - ➤ Antiplatelet medicines and blood-thinning medicines, such as aspirin. These help prevent blood clots.
  - ➤ Medicine that dissolves any blood clots (*fibrinolytic therapy*).
  - ➤ Blood pressure medicines.
  - ➤ Nitroglycerin. This helps widen blood vessels to improve blood flow.
  - ➤ Pain medicine.
  - ➤ Cholesterol-lowering medicine.

  - Surgery, such as:
    - ➤ Coronary angioplasty with stent placement. This involves placing a small piece of metal that looks like mesh or a spring into a narrow coronary artery. This widens the artery and keeps it open.
    - ➤ Coronary artery bypass surgery. This involves taking a section of a blood vessel from a different part of your body and placing it on the blocked coronary artery to allow blood to flow around the blockage.

- Cardiac rehabilitation. This is a program that includes exercise training, education, and counseling to help you recover.

# Follow these instructions at home:

## Eating and drinking

- Eat a heart-healthy diet that includes whole grains, fruits and vegetables, lean proteins, and low-fat or nonfat dairy products.
- Limit how much salt (*sodium*) you eat as told by your health care provider. Follow instructions from your health care provider about any other eating or drinking restrictions, such as limiting foods that are high in fat and processed sugars.
- Use healthy cooking methods such as roasting, grilling, broiling, baking, poaching, steaming, or stir-frying.
- Work with a dietitian to follow a heart-healthy eating plan.

## Medicines

- Take over-the-counter and prescription medicines only as told by your health care provider.
- **Do not** take these medicines unless your health care provider approves:
  - Vitamin supplements that contain vitamin A or vitamin E.
  - NSAIDs, such as ibuprofen, naproxen, or celecoxib.
  - Hormone replacement therapy that contains estrogen.
- If you are taking blood thinners:
  - Talk with your health care provider before you take any medicines that contain aspirin or NSAIDs. These medicines increase your risk for dangerous bleeding.
  - Take your medicine exactly as told, at the same time every day.
  - Avoid activities that could cause injury or bruising, and follow instructions about how to prevent falls.

> Wear a medical alert bracelet, and carry a card that lists what medicines you take.

## Activity

- Follow your cardiac rehabilitation program. Do exercises as told by your physical therapist.
- Ask your health care provider what activities and exercises are safe for you. Follow his or her instructions about lifting, driving, or climbing stairs.

## Lifestyle

- **Do not** use any products that contain nicotine or tobacco, such as cigarettes, e-cigarettes, and chewing tobacco. If you need help quitting, ask your health care provider.
- **Do not** drink alcohol if your health care provider tells you not to drink.
- If you drink alcohol:
  > Limit how much you have to 0–1 drink a day.
  > Be aware of how much alcohol is in your drink. In the U.S., one drink equals one 12 oz bottle of beer (355 mL), one 5 oz glass of wine (148 mL), or one 1½ oz glass of hard liquor (44 mL).
- Maintain a healthy weight. If you need to lose weight, work with your health care provider to do so safely.

# General instructions

- Tell all the health care providers who provide care for you about your heart condition, including your dentist. This may affect the medicines or treatment you receive.
- Manage any other health conditions you have, such as hypertension or diabetes. These conditions affect your heart.

- Pay attention to your mental health. You may be at higher risk for depression.

  ➢ Find ways to manage stress.
  ➢ Talk to your health care provider about depression screening and treatment.

- Keep your vaccinations up to date.

  ➢ Get the flu shot (*influenza vaccine*) every year.
  ➢ Get the pneumococcal vaccine if you are age 65 or older.

- If directed, monitor your blood pressure at home.
- Keep all follow-up visits as told by your health care provider. This is important.

## Contact a health care provider if you:

- Feel overwhelmed or sad.
- Have trouble doing your daily activities.

## Get help right away if you:

- Have pain in your chest, neck, arm, jaw, stomach, or back that recurs, and:

  ➢ It lasts for more than a few minutes.
  ➢ It is not relieved by taking the medicineyour health care provider prescribed.

- Have unexplained:

  ➢ Heavy sweating.
  ➢ Heartburn or indigestion.
  ➢ Nausea or vomiting.
  ➢ Shortness of breath.
  ➢ Difficulty breathing.
  ➢ Fatigue.

- Nervousness or anxiety.
- Weakness.
- Diarrhea.
- Dark stools or blood in your stool.

- Have sudden light-headedness or dizziness.
- Have blood pressure that is higher than 180/120.
- Faint.
- Have thoughts about hurting yourself.

**These symptoms may represent a serious problem that is an emergency. Do not wait to see if the symptoms will go away. Get medical help right away. Call your local emergency services (911 in the U.S.). Do not drive yourself to the hospital.**

## Summary

- Acute coronary syndrome (ACS) is when there is not enough blood and oxygen being supplied to the heart. ACS can result in chest pain or a heart attack.
- Acute coronary syndrome is a medical emergency. If you have any symptoms of this condition, get help right away.
- Treatment includes medicines and procedures to open the blocked arteries and restore blood flow.

This information is not intended to replace advice given to you by your health care provider. Make sure you discuss any questions you have with your health care provider.

# Angina

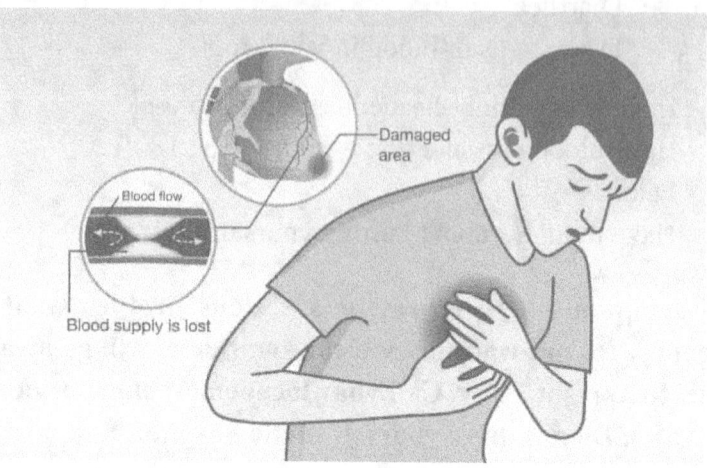

Angina is extreme discomfort in the chest, neck, arm, jaw, or back. The discomfort is caused by a lack of blood in the middle layer of the heart wall (*myocardium*).

There are four types of angina:

- Stable angina. This is triggered by vigorous activity or exercise. It goes away when you rest or take angina medicine.
- Unstable angina. This is a warning sign and can lead to a heart attack (*acute coronary syndrome*). **This is a medical emergency.** Symptoms come at rest and last a long time.
- Microvascular angina. This affects the small coronary arteries. Symptoms include feeling tired and being short of breath.
- Prinzmetal or variant angina. This is caused by a tightening (*spasm*) of the arteries that go to your heart.

# What are the causes?

This condition is caused by atherosclerosis. This is the buildup of fat and cholesterol (*plaque*) in your arteries. The plaque may narrow or block the artery.

Other causes of angina include:

- Sudden tightening of the muscles of the arteries in the heart (*coronary spasm*).
- Small artery disease (*microvascular dysfunction*).
- Problems with any of your heart valves (*heart valve disease*).
- A tear in an artery in your heart (*coronary artery dissection*).
- Diseases of the heart muscle (*cardiomyopathy*), or other heart diseases.

# What increases the risk?

You are more likely to develop this condition if you have:

- High cholesterol.
- High blood pressure (*hypertension*).
- Diabetes.
- A family history of heart disease.
- An inactive (*sedentary*) lifestyle, or you do not exercise enough.
- Depression.
- Had radiation treatment to the left side of your chest.

Other risk factors include:

- Using tobacco.
- Being obese.
- Eating a diet high in saturated fats.

- Being exposed to high stress or triggers of stress.
- Using drugs, such as cocaine.

Women have a greater risk for angina if:

- They are older than 55.
- They have gone through menopause (are *postmenopausal*).

## What are the signs or symptoms?

Common symptoms of this condition in both men and women may include:

- Chest pain, which may:

  ➢ Feel like a crushing or squeezing in the chest, or like a tightness, pressure, fullness, or heaviness in the chest.
  ➢ Last for more than a few minutes at a time, or it may stop and come back (*recur*) over the course of a few minutes.

- Pain in the neck, arm, jaw, or back.
- Unexplained heartburn or indigestion.
- Shortness of breath.
- Nausea.
- Sudden cold sweats.

Women and people with diabetes may have unusual (*atypical*) symptoms, such as:

- Fatigue.
- Unexplained feelings of nervousness or anxiety.
- Unexplained weakness.
- Dizziness or fainting.

# How is this diagnosed?

This condition may be diagnosed based on:

- Your symptoms and medical history.
- Electrocardiogram (ECG) to measure the electrical activity in your heart.
- Blood tests.
- Stress test to look for signs of blockage when your heart is stressed.
- CT angiogram to examine your heart and the blood flow to it.
- Coronary angiogram to check your coronary arteries for blockage.

# How is this treated?

Angina may be treated with:

- Medicines to:
  - Prevent blood clots and heart attack.
  - Relax blood vessels and improve blood flow to the heart (*nitrates*).
  - Reduce blood pressure, improve the pumping action of the heart, and relax blood vessels that are spasming.
  - Reduce cholesterol and help treat atherosclerosis.

- A procedure to widen a narrowed or blocked coronary artery (*angioplasty*). A mesh tube may be placed in a coronary artery to keep it open (*coronary stenting*).
- Surgery to allow blood to go around a blocked artery (*coronary artery bypass surgery*).

# Follow these instructions at home:

## Medicines

- Take over-the-counter and prescription medicines only as told by your health care provider.
- **Do not** take the following medicines unless your health care provider approves:

  ➢ NSAIDs, such as ibuprofen or naproxen.
  ➢ Vitamin supplements that contain vitamin A, vitamin E, or both.
  ➢ Hormone replacement therapy that contains estrogen with or without progestin.

## Eating and drinking

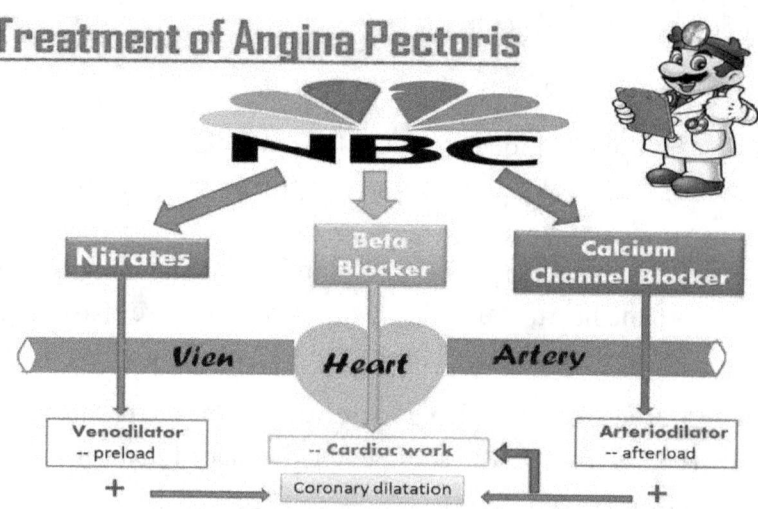

- Eat a heart-healthy diet. This includes plenty of fresh fruits and vegetables, whole grains, low-fat (*lean*) protein, and low-fat dairy products.

- Follow instructions from your health care provider about eating or drinking restrictions.

## Activity

- Follow an exercise program approved by your health care provider.
- Consider joining a cardiac rehabilitation program.
- Take a break when you feel fatigued. Plan rest periods in your daily activities.

## Lifestyle

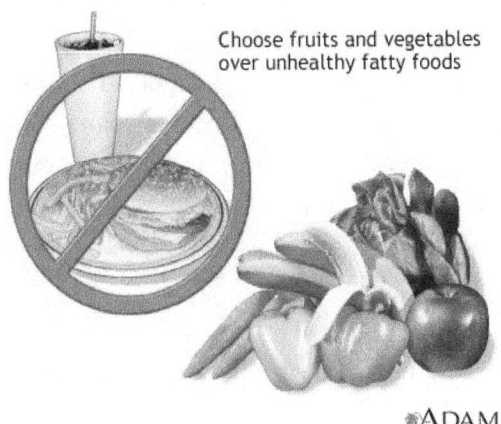

Choose fruits and vegetables over unhealthy fatty foods

⬧ADAM.

- **Do not** use any products that contain nicotine or tobacco, such as cigarettes, e-cigarettes, and chewing tobacco. If you need help quitting, ask your health care provider.
- If your health care provider says you can drink alcohol:

  ➢ Limit how much you use to:

    o 0–1 drink a day for non-pregnant women.
    o 0–2 drinks a day for men.

41

➤ Be aware of how much alcohol is in your drink. In the U.S., one drink equals one 12 oz bottle of beer (355 mL), one 5 oz glass of wine (148 mL), or one 1½ oz glass of hard liquor (44 mL).

## General instructions

- Maintain a healthy weight.
- Learn to manage stress.
- Keep your vaccinations up to date. Get the flu (*influenza*) vaccine every year.
- Talk to your health care provider if you feel depressed. Take a depression screening test to see if you are at risk for depression.
- Work with your health care provider to manage other health conditions, such as hypertension or diabetes.
- Keep all follow-up visits as told by your health care provider. This is important.

## Get help right away if:

- You have pain in your chest, neck, arm, jaw, or back, and the pain:
  - ➤ Lasts more than a few minutes.
  - ➤ Is recurring.
  - ➤ Is not relieved by taking medicines under the tongue (*sublingual nitroglycerin*).
  - ➤ Increases in intensity or frequency.
- You have a lot of sweating without cause.
- You have unexplained:
  - ➤ Heartburn or indigestion.
  - ➤ Shortness of breath or difficulty breathing.
  - ➤ Nausea or vomiting.

- ➤ Fatigue.
- ➤ Feelings of nervousness or anxiety.
- ➤ Weakness.

- You have sudden light-headedness or dizziness.
- You faint.

**These symptoms may represent a serious problem that is an emergency. Do not wait to see if the symptoms will go away. Get medical help right away. Call your local emergency services (911 in the U.S.). Do not drive yourself to the hospital.**

## Summary

- Angina is extreme discomfort in the chest, neck, arm, jaw, or back that is caused by a lack of blood in the heart wall.
- There are many symptoms of angina. They include chest pain, unexplained heartburn or indigestion, sudden cold sweats, and fatigue.
- Angina may be treated with behavioral changes, medicine, or surgery.
- Symptoms of angina may represent an emergency. Get medical help right away. Call your local emergency services (911 in the U.S.). **Do not** drive yourself to the hospital.

This information is not intended to replace advice given to you by your health care provider. Make sure you discuss any questions you have with your health care provider.

**These symptoms may represent a serious problem that is an emergency. Do not wait to see if the symptoms will go away. Get medical help right away. Call your local emergency services (911 in the U.S.). Do not drive yourself to the hospital.**

# Summary

- Atherosclerosis is narrowing and hardening of the arteries.
- Arteries can become narrow or clogged with a buildup of fat, cholesterol, calcium, and other substances (plaque).
- This condition may not cause any symptoms. If you do have symptoms, they are caused by damage to an area of your body that is not getting enough blood.
- Treatment may include lifestyle changes and medicines. In some cases, surgery is needed

# Coronary Microvascular Disease

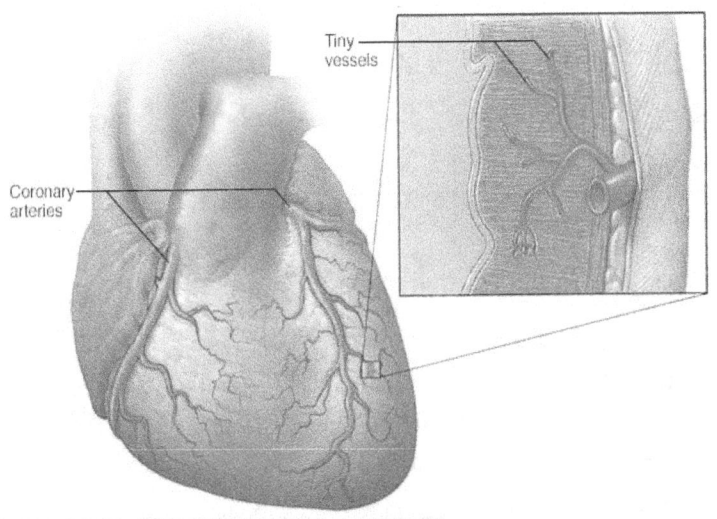

Tiny vessels

Coronary arteries

Coronary microvascular disease (MVD) is a heart (*coronary*) disease in which the walls and inner lining of the heart's small arteries are damaged. The damage may lead to a tightening (*spasm*) of the arteries, which causes decreased blood flow to the heart. This is different from coronary artery disease (CAD), in which plaque builds up in the large arteries of the heart. The risk factors for MVD are similar to those for CAD, and microvascular disease is more common in women.

## What are the causes?

Common causes of this condition include:

- High blood pressure.
- Diabetes.
- Smoking.
- High cholesterol.
- Being overweight or obese.

- Inactivity (*sedentary lifestyle*).
- Unhealthy diet.
- Family history of early heart disease.
- Being a female.
- Having anxiety or depression.

The causes of MVD are also considered to be risk factors for MVD.

## What are the signs or symptoms?

Symptoms of this condition include:

- Chest pain (*angina*). This may feel like a burning, squeezing, or pressure sensation. It can spread (*radiate*) to the neck, arm, back, or jaw. Angina usually lasts at least 10 minutes and can last longer than 30 minutes.
- Shortness of breath.
- Nausea.
- Weakness.
- Dizziness.
- Sweating
- Fluttering or fast heartbeat (*palpitations*).
- Sleep problems.
- Fatigue.
- Lack of energy.

People often notice their first symptoms of MVD during their routine daily activities and at times of mental stress. Symptoms are often less noticeable during physical activity.

## How is this diagnosed?

This condition may be diagnosed based on:

- Your medical history.
- Your symptoms.

- A physical exam.
- Blood tests.
- Electrocardiogram (ECG). This test checks the electrical activity in the heart.
- PET scan of the heart (*cardiac PET scan*). This imaging test makes pictures to show healthy and damaged heart muscle.
- MRI of the heart (*cardiac MRI*). This imaging test shows the function and structure of the heart and blood vessels (*cardiovascular system*).
- An exercise stress test. For this test, your heart function and blood pressure are monitored before, during, and after exercise. An ECG is used during this test.
- Coronary angiogram with additional blood flow testing. For this procedure, dye is injected into your coronary arteries before X-rays are taken to check blood flow and heart function.

Sometimes, standard tests do not show MVD. Standard coronary angiogram only shows blockages in the large arteries. You may still be diagnosed with MVD, even if the angiogram results are normal.

## How is this treated?

This condition is managed with medicines, such as:

- Medicines to control cholesterol levels (*statins*).
- Medicines to lower blood pressure (*ACE inhibitors* or *beta blockers*).
- Aspirin to prevent blood clots or to control inflammation.
- Medicine to treat angina and improve blood flow to the heart (*nitroglycerin*).

# Follow these instructions at home:

### Lifestyle

- Be physically active every day. Ask your health care provider how much physical activity you need and what types of exercise are best for you.
- **Do not** use any products that contain nicotine or tobacco, such as cigarettes and e-cigarettes. If you need help quitting, ask your health care provider.
- Follow a heart-healthy diet. A diet and nutrition specialist (*dietitian*) can help you learn about healthy food options and changes. In general, eat plenty of fruits and vegetables, lean meats, and whole grains.

## General instructions

- Take over-the-counter and prescription medicines only as told by your health care provider.
- If you are overweight or obese, work with your health care provider to lose weight safely.
- Manage any other health conditions that affect your heart, such as hypertension and diabetes.
- Keep all follow-up visits as told by your health care provider. This is important.

## Contact a health care provider if:

- You have chest pain.
- You have trouble doing your daily activities.

## Get help right away if:

- You have discomfort in the center of your chest that:

> Lasts for more than a few minutes.
> Goes away and comes back (*recurs*).

- You have shortness of breath.
- You have pressure, pain, or a sense of fullness or squeezing in your chest.
- You feel nauseous.
- You feel light-headed.
- You have chills.

**These symptoms may represent a serious problem that is an emergency. Do not wait to see if the symptoms will go away. Get medical help right away. Call your local emergency services (911 in the U.S.). Do not drive yourself to the hospital.**

## Summary

- Coronary microvascular disease (MVD) is a heart (*coronary*) disease in which the walls and inner lining of the heart's small arteries are damaged.
- Symptoms of this condition include chest pain (*angina*). This usually lasts at least 10 minutes and can last longer than 30 minutes.
- This condition is diagnosed by your health care provider based on your medical history, a physical exam, and test results.
- This condition is managed with medicines and other lifestyle changes.

This information is not intended to replace advice given to you by your health care provider. Make sure you discuss any questions you have with your health care provider

# Heart Disease Prevention

Heart disease is the leading cause of death in the world. Coronary artery disease is the most common cause of heart disease. This condition results when cholesterol and other substances (*plaque*) build up inside the walls of the blood vessels that supply your heart muscle (*arteries*). This buildup in arteries is called atherosclerosis. You can take actions to lower your risk of heart disease.

## How can heart disease affect me?

Heart disease can cause many unpleasant symptoms and complications, such as:

- Chest pain (*angina*).
- Reduced or blocked blood flow to your heart. This can cause:
  - ➤ Irregular heartbeats (*arrhythmias*).
  - ➤ Heart attack.
  - ➤ Heart failure.

## What can increase my risk?

The following factors may make you more likely to develop this condition:

- High blood pressure (*hypertension*).
- High cholesterol.
- Smoking.
- A diet high in saturated fats or *trans* fats.
- Lack of physical activity.
- Obesity.
- Drinking too much alcohol.
- Diabetes.
- Having a family history of heart disease.

# What actions can I take to prevent heart disease?

## Nutrition

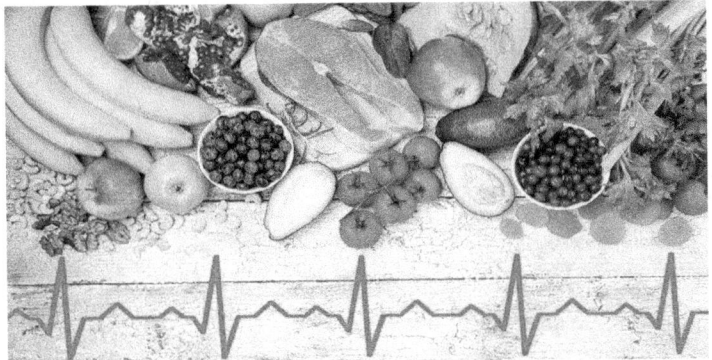

- Eat a heart-healthy eating plan as told by your health care provider. Examples include the DASH (Dietary Approaches to Stop Hypertension) eating plan or the Mediterranean diet.
- Generally, it is recommended that you:
  - ➤ Eat less salt (*sodium*). Ask your health care provider how much sodium is safe for you. Most people should have less than 2,300 mg each day.
  - ➤ Limit unhealthy fats, such as saturated and *trans* fats, in your diet. You can do this by eating low-fat dairy products, eating less red meat, and avoiding processed foods.
  - ➤ Eat healthy fats (*omega-3 fatty acids*). These are found in fish, such as mackerel or salmon.
  - ➤ Eat more fruits and vegetables. You should try to fill one-half of your plate with fruits and vegetables at each meal.
  - ➤ Eat more whole grains.
  - ➤ Avoid foods and drinks that have added sugars.

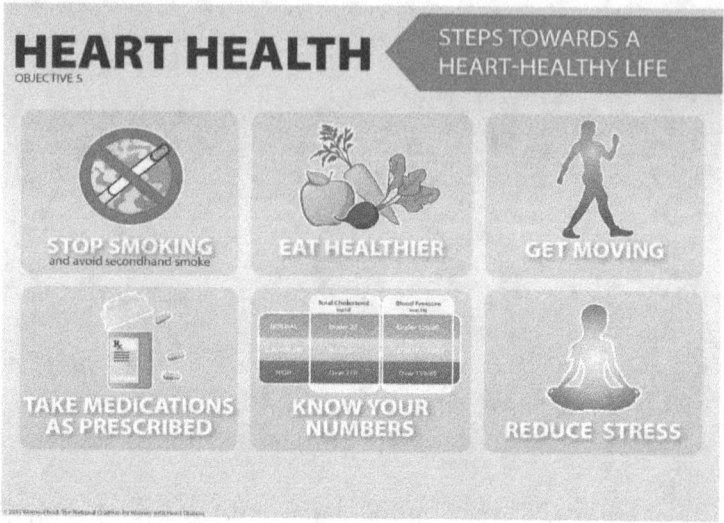

- Get regular exercise. This is one of the most important things you can do for your health. Generally, it is recommended that you:

  - Exercise for at least 30 minutes on most days of the week (150 minutes each week). The exercise should increase your heart rate and make you sweat (*aerobic exercise*).
  - Add strength exercises on at least 2 days each week.

- **Do not** use any products that contain nicotine or tobacco, such as cigarettes and e-cigarettes. These can damage your heart and blood vessels. If you need help quitting, ask your health care provider.

## Alcohol use

- **Do not** drink alcohol if:

  - Your health care provider tells you not to drink.

- You are pregnant, may be pregnant, or are planning to become pregnant.
- If you drink alcohol, limit how much you have:
  - 0–1 drink a day for women.
  - 0–2 drinks a day for men.
- Be aware of how much alcohol is in your drink. In the U.S., one drink equals one typical bottle of beer (12 oz), one-half glass of wine (5 oz), or one shot of hard liquor (1½ oz).

## Medicines

- Take over-the-counter and prescription medicines only as told by your health care provider.
- Ask your health care provider whether you should take an aspirin every day. Taking aspirin may help reduce your risk of heart disease and stroke.
- Depending on your risk factors, your health care provider may prescribe medicines to lower your risk of heart disease or to control related conditions. You may take medicine to:
  - Lower cholesterol.
  - Control blood pressure.
  - Control diabetes.

## General information

- Keep your blood pressure under control, as recommended by your health care provider. For most healthy people, the upper number of your blood pressure (*systolic*) should be no higher than 120, and the lower number (*diastolic*) no higher than 80. Treatment may be needed if your blood pressure is higher than 130/80.

- Have your blood pressure checked at least every two years. Your health care provider may check your blood pressure more often if you have high blood pressure.
- After age 20, have your cholesterol checked every 4–6 years. If you have risk factors for heart disease, you may need to have it checked more frequently. Treatment may be needed if your cholesterol is high.
- Have your body mass index (BMI) checked every year. Your health care provider can calculate your BMI from your height and weight.
- Work with your health care provider to lose weight, if needed, or to maintain a healthy weight.

## Where to find more information:

- Centers for Disease Control and Prevention: www.cdc.gov/heartdisease
- American Heart Association: www.heart.org

  ➢ Take a free online heart disease risk quiz to better understand your personal risk factors.

## Summary

- Heart disease is the leading cause of death in the world.
- Heart disease can cause chest pain, abnormal heart rhythms, heart attack, and heart failure.
- High blood pressure, high cholesterol, and smoking are the main risk factors for heart disease, although other factors also contribute.
- You can take actions to lower your chances of developing heart disease. Work with your health care provider to reduce your risk by following a heart-healthy diet, being physically active, and controlling your weight, blood pressure, and cholesterol level.

This information is not intended to replace advice given to you by your health care provider. Make sure you discuss any questions you have with your health care provider.

## Cardiac CT Angiogram

A cardiac CT angiogram is a procedure to look at the heart and the area around the heart. It may be done to help find the cause of chest pains or other symptoms of heart disease. During this procedure, a substance called contrast dye is injected into the blood vessels in the area to be checked. A large X-ray machine, called a CT scanner, then takes detailed pictures of the heart and the surrounding area. The procedure is also sometimes called a coronary CT angiogram, coronary artery scanning, or CTA.

A cardiac CT angiogram allows the health care provider to see how well blood is flowing to and from the heart. The health care provider will be able to see if there are any problems, such as:

- Blockage or narrowing of the coronary arteries in the heart.
- Fluid around the heart.
- Signs of weakness or disease in the muscles, valves, and tissues of the heart.

## Tell a health care provider about:

- Any allergies you have. This is especially important if you have had a previous allergic reaction to contrast dye.
- All medicines you are taking, including vitamins, herbs, eye drops, creams, and over-the-counter medicines.
- Any blood disorders you have.
- Any surgeries you have had.
- Any medical conditions you have.
- Whether you are pregnant or may be pregnant.

- Any anxiety disorders, chronic pain, or other conditions you have that may increase your stress or prevent you from lying still.

## What are the risks?

Generally, this is a safe procedure. However, problems may occur, including:

- Bleeding.
- Infection.
- Allergic reactions to medicines or dyes.
- Damage to other structures or organs.
- Kidney damage from the contrast dye that is used.
- Increased risk of cancer from radiation exposure. This risk is low. Talk with your health care provider about:

  ➢ The risks and benefits of testing.
  ➢ How you can receive the lowest dose of radiation.

## What happens before the procedure?

- Wear comfortable clothing and remove any jewelry, glasses, dentures, and hearing aids.
- Follow instructions from your health care provider about eating and drinking. This may include:

  ➢ For 12 hours before the procedure — avoid caffeine. This includes tea, coffee, soda, energy drinks, and diet pills. Drink plenty of water or other fluids that do not have caffeine in them. Being well hydrated can prevent complications.
  ➢ For 4–6 hours before the procedure — stop eating and drinking. The contrast dye can cause nausea, but this is less likely if your stomach is empty.

- Ask your health care provider about changing or stopping your regular medicines. This is especially important if you are taking diabetes medicines, blood thinners, or medicines to treat problems with erections (*erectile dysfunction*).

## What happens during the procedure?

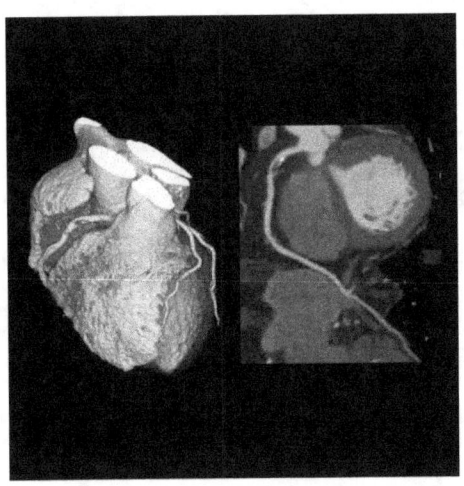

- Hair on your chest may need to be removed so that small sticky patches called electrodes can be placed on your chest. These will transmit information that helps to monitor your heart during the procedure.
- An IV will be inserted into one of your veins.
- You might be given a medicine to control your heart rate during the procedure. This will help to ensure that good images are obtained.
- You will be asked to lie on an exam table. This table will slide in and out of the CT machine during the procedure.
- Contrast dye will be injected into the IV. You might feel warm, or you may get a metallic taste in your mouth.
- You will be given a medicine called nitroglycerin. This will relax or dilate the arteries in your heart.

- The table that you are lying on will move into the CT machine tunnel for the scan.
- The person running the machine will give you instructions while the scans are being done. You may be asked to:
  - ➢ Keep your arms above your head.
  - ➢ Hold your breath.
  - ➢ Stay very still, even if the table is moving.
- When the scanning is complete, you will be moved out of the machine.
- The IV will be removed.

The procedure may vary among health care providers and hospitals.

## What can I expect after the procedure?

After your procedure, it is common to have:

- A metallic taste in your mouth from the contrast dye.
- A feeling of warmth.
- A headache from the nitroglycerin.

## Follow these instructions at home:

- Take over-the-counter and prescription medicines only as told by your health care provider.
- If you are told, drink enough fluid to keep your urine pale yellow. This will help to flush the contrast dye out of your body.
- Most people can return to their normal activities right after the procedure. Ask your health care provider what activities are safe for you.
- It is up to you to get the results of your procedure. Ask your health care provider, or the department that is doing the procedure, when your results will be ready.

- Keep all follow-up visits as told by your health care provider. This is important.

## Contact a health care provider if:

- You have any symptoms of allergy to the contrast dye. These include:
  - ➤ Shortness of breath.
  - ➤ Rash or hives.
  - ➤ A racing heartbeat.

## Summary

- A cardiac CT angiogram is a procedure to look at the heart and the area around the heart. It may be done to help find the cause of chest pains or other symptoms of heart disease.
- During this procedure, a large X-ray machine, called a CT scanner, takes detailed pictures of the heart and the surrounding area after a contrast dye has been injected into blood vessels in the area.
- Ask your health care provider about changing or stopping your regular medicines before the procedure. This is especially important if you are taking diabetes medicines, blood thinners, or medicines to treat erectile dysfunction.
- If you are told, drink enough fluid to keep your urine pale yellow. This will help to flush the contrast dye out of your body.

This information is not intended to replace advice given to you by your health care provider. Make sure you discuss any questions you have with your health care provider

# Atherectomy

An atherectomy is a surgical procedure to remove a buildup of fat, cholesterol, and other substances (*plaque*) from the inside of an artery. Arteries are the blood vessels that carry blood from the heart to the rest of the body. A buildup of plaque in the arteries can block blood flow. In this procedure, plaque is removed from an artery using a device at the end of a thin, flexible tube (*catheter*). A narrow tube of wire mesh (*stent*) may be placed in the artery to prevent it from getting blocked again.

You may have this procedure to remove plaque from the arteries of your heart (*coronary arteries*). You can also have this procedure to clear arteries in other parts of your body, such as the arteries that provide blood to your legs.

## Tell a health care provider about:

- Any allergies you have.
- All medicines you are taking, including vitamins, herbs, eye drops, creams, and over-the-counter medicines.
- Any problems you or family members have had with anesthetic medicines.
- Any blood disorders you have.
- Any surgeries you have had.
- Any medical conditions you have.
- Whether you are pregnant or may be pregnant.

## What are the risks?

Generally, this is a safe procedure. However, problems may occur, including:

- Infection.
- Bleeding.

- Allergic reactions to medicines or dyes.
- Damage to other structures or organs.
- Inability to open the blocked artery.
- Artery rupture.
- Heart attack (if the procedure is done on a heart artery).
- Amputation (if the procedure is done on a leg artery).
- Return of the blockage or clotting.
- A blood clot that can lead to a stroke.

## What happens before the procedure?

- Ask your health care provider about:
  - ➢ Changing or stopping your regular medicines. This is especially important if you are taking diabetes medicines or blood thinners.
  - ➢ Taking medicines such as aspirin and ibuprofen. These medicines can thin your blood. **Do not** take these medicines unless your health care provider tells you to take them.
  - ➢ Taking over-the-counter medicines, vitamins, herbs, and supplements.
- Follow instructions from your health care provider about eating or drinking restrictions.
- Plan to have someone take you home from the hospital or clinic.
- Plan to have a responsible adult care for you for at least 24 hours after you leave the hospital or clinic. This is important.
- You may be given antibiotic medicine to help prevent an infection.
- You may be asked to shower with a germ-killing soap.

# What happens during the procedure?

- To lower your risk of infection:

  ➤ Your health care team will wash or sanitize their hands.
  ➤ Hair may be removed from your groin area.
  ➤ Your skin will be washed with soap.

- An IV will be inserted into one of your veins.
- Sticky patches (*electrodes*) will be placed on your chest to monitor your heart rhythm.
- You will be given one or more of the following:

  ➤ A medicine to help you relax (*sedative*).
  ➤ A medicine to numb the groin or wrist area (*local anesthetic*).

- Your health care provider will make a small incision in your groin area or wrist and identify the needed artery.
- A catheter will be put into the artery and guided to the location of the plaque. Your health care provider will use X-ray images to guide the catheter to the right spot.
- Dye will be injected into the artery after the catheter is in the correct position.
- Your health care provider will use an instrument that is inserted through the catheter to cut away pieces of plaque. The pieces will be stored in part of the catheter so they can be removed.
- A stent will likely be put in place to keep your artery open.
- The catheter will be removed.
- The incision will be closed and covered with a certain type of bandage (*pressure dressing*).

The procedure may vary among health care providers and hospitals.

# What happens after the procedure?

- Your blood pressure, heart rate, breathing rate, and blood oxygen level will be monitored until the medicines you were given have worn off.
- After several hours, you will be encouraged to get up and walk around.
- **Do not** drive for 24 hours if you were given a sedative during your procedure.

# Summary

- An atherectomy is a surgical procedure to remove a buildup of fat, cholesterol, and other substances (*plaque*) from the inside of an artery.
- In this procedure, plaque is removed from an artery using a device at the end of a thin, flexible tube (*catheter*). A narrow tube of wire mesh (*stent*) will likely be placed in the artery to prevent it from getting blocked again.
- Before the procedure, ask your health care provider about changing or stopping your regular medicines. Also follow any instructions about eating or drinking restrictions.

This information is not intended to replace advice given to you by your health care provider. Make sure you discuss any questions you have with your health care provids you have with

## Atherectomy, Care After

This sheet gives you information about how to care for yourself after your procedure. Your health care provider may also give you more specific instructions. If you have problems or questions, contact your health care provider.

# What can I expect after the procedure?

After the procedure, it is common to have:

- A tender lump in your groin or wrist.
- Bruising.
- Soreness.

# Follow these instructions at home:

## Incision site care

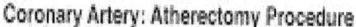

Coronary Artery: Atherectomy Procedure

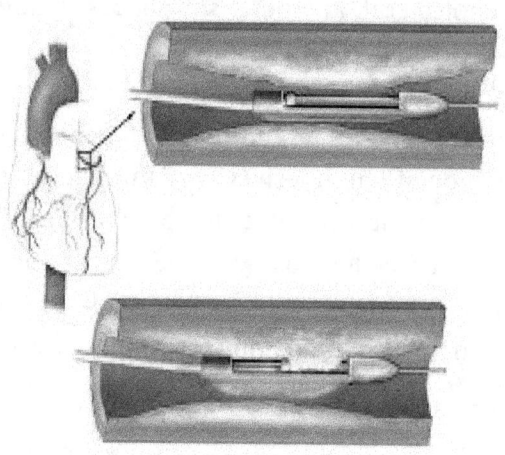

- Follow instructions from your health care provider about how to take care of your incision. Make sure you:
  - ➢ Wash your hands with soap and water before you change your bandage (*dressing*). If soap and water are not available, use hand sanitizer.
  - ➢ Change your dressing as told by your health care provider.

- ➢ Leave stitches (*sutures*), skin glue, or adhesive strips in place. These skin closures may need to stay in place for 2 weeks or longer. If adhesive strip edges start to loosen and curl up, you may trim the loose edges. **Do not** remove adhesive strips completely unless your health care provider tells you to do that.
- Check your incision area every day for signs of infection. Check for:
  - ➢ Redness, swelling, or pain.
  - ➢ Fluid or blood.
  - ➢ Warmth.
  - ➢ Pus or a bad smell.
- **Do not** take baths, swim, or use a hot tub until your health care provider approves. Ask your health care provider if you may take showers.

## Activity

- Return to your normal activities as told by your health care provider. Ask your health care provider what activities are safe for you.
- **Do not** lift anything that is heavier than 10 lb (4.5 kg), or the limit that you are told, until your health care provider says that it is safe.
- **Do not** drive for 24 hours if you were given a medicine to help you relax (*sedative*) during your procedure.

## Lifestyle

- Make any lifestyle changes as recommended by your health care provider. These may include:

- Not using any products that contain nicotine or tobacco, such as cigarettes and e-cigarettes. If you need help quitting, ask your health care provider.
- Managing your weight.
- Getting exercise on a regular basis.
- Managing your blood pressure.
- Limiting your alcohol intake.
- Managing other health problems, such as diabetes.

- Eat a healthy diet. This should include plenty of fresh fruits and vegetables. Avoid foods that are:
  - High in salt (*sodium*).
  - Canned or highly processed.
  - High in saturated fat or sugar.
  - Fried.

## General instructions

- Take over-the-counter and prescription medicines only as told by your health care provider.
- Drink enough fluid to keep your urine pale yellow.
- Keep all follow-up visits as told by your health care provider. This is important.

## Contact a health care provider if:

- You have a fever or chills.
- You have redness, swelling, or pain around your incision.
- You have fluid or blood coming from your incision.
- Your incision area feels warm to the touch.
- You have pus or a bad smell coming from your incision.

# Get help right away if:

- You have uncontrolled bleeding at your incision site.
- You have chest pain.
- You have trouble breathing.
- Your toes are blue, discolored, or painful.

# Summary

- After the procedure, it is common to have soreness, bruising, or a tender lump in your groin or wrist where the catheter was inserted.
- Return to your normal activities as told by your health care provider. Ask your health care provider what activities are safe for you.
- Follow instructions from your health care provider about how to take care of your incision. Check your incision area every day for signs of infection.
- This information is not intended to replace advice given to you by your health care provider. Make sure you discuss any question

## Apolipoproteins Test

# Why am I having this test?

The apolipoproteins test is ordered to evaluate a person's risk for coronary artery disease (CAD) and high cholesterol by looking at several indicators.

# What is being tested?

The test may include measurements of the following:

- Apolipoprotein A-1 (Apo A-1). This is an indicator of high-density lipoprotein (HDL) cholesterol. Low levels of HDL are a risk factor for CAD.
- Apolipoprotein B (Apo B). This is an indicator of low-density lipoprotein (LDL) cholesterol and very-low-density lipoprotein (VLDL) cholesterol. High levels of LDL and VLDL are risk factors for CAD.
- Lipoprotein (a) [Lp(a)]. This is an indicator of LDL-like proteins. High levels are considered a risk factor for CAD.
- Apolipoprotein E (Apo E). This is involved in cholesterol transport in the body. Certain forms of the Apo E gene are associated with high cholesterol, high LDL, and increased risk for Alzheimer's disease.

## What kind of sample is taken?

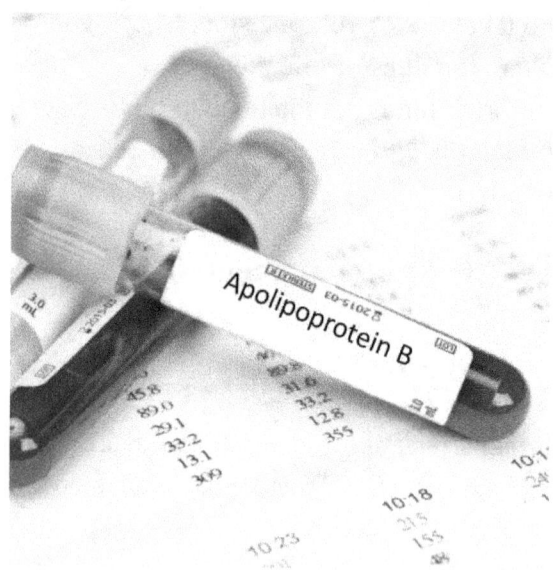

A blood sample is required for this test. It is usually collected by inserting a needle into a blood vessel.

# How do I prepare for this test?

Your health care provider may instruct you not to eat or drink for 12–14 hours before your test. Water is permitted. You may also be asked to stop smoking for a period of time before the test.

# How are the results reported?

Your test results will be reported as values. Your health care provider will compare your results to normal ranges that were established after testing a large group of people (*reference ranges*). Reference ranges may vary among labs and hospitals. For this test, common reference ranges are:

- **Apo A-1**
  - ➢ Adult/elderly:
    - ○ Male: 75–160 mg/dL.
    - ○ Female: 80–175 mg/dL.

  - ➢ 5–17 years: 83–151 mg/dL.

  - ➢ 6 months–4 years:
    - ○ Male: 67–167 mg/dL.
    - ○ Female: 60–148 mg/dL.

  - ➢ Newborn:
    - ○ Male: 41–93 mg/dL.
    - ○ Female: 38–106 mg/dL.

- **Apo B**
  - ➢ Adult/elderly:
    - ○ Male: 50–125 mg/dL.

- o Female: 45–120 mg/dL.

  - ➤ 5–17 years:
    - o Male: 47–139 mg/dL.
    - o Female: 41–132 mg/dL.

  - ➤ 6 months–3 years: 23–75 mg/dL.

  - ➤ Newborn: 11–31 mg/dL.

- **Apo A-1/Apo B ratio**
  - ➤ Male: 0.85–2.24.
  - ➤ Female: 0.76–3.23.

- **Lp(a)**
  - ➤ Caucasian (5th–95th percentile):
    - o Male: 2.2–49.4 mg/dL.
    - o Female: 2.1–57.3 mg/dL.

  - ➤ African American (5th–95th percentile):
    - o Male: 4.6–71.8 mg/dL.
    - o Female: 4.4–75 mg/dL.

- **Apo E**
  - ➤ Apo E genotyping results are reported as either positive or negative for the different gene forms.

## What do the results mean?

- Decreased levels of Apo A-1 are associated with an increased risk for CAD.
- Increased levels of Apo B are associated with an increased risk for CAD.

- Increased levels of Lp(a) are associated with an increased risk for CAD.
- A positive test for certain forms of the Apo E gene are associated with high cholesterol, high LDL, and increased risk for Alzheimer's disease.
- Many other conditions are known to be associated with increased and decreased levels of apolipoproteins.

Talk with your health care provider about what your results mean.

## Questions to ask your health care provider

Ask your health care provider, or the department that is doing the test:

- When will my results be ready?
- How will I get my results?
- What are my treatment options?
- What other tests do I need?
- What are my next steps?

## Summary

- The apolipoproteins test is ordered to evaluate a person's risk for coronary artery disease (CAD) and high cholesterol by looking at several indicators.
- You may be asked not to smoke, eat, or drink anything (except water) for 12–14 hours before your blood sample is collected.
- Talk with your health care provider about what your results mean.

This information is not intended to replace advice given to you by your health care provider. Make sure you discuss any questions you have with your health care provider.

# Coronary Calcium Scan

A coronary calcium scan is an imaging test used to look for deposits of plaque in the inner lining of the blood vessels of the heart (*coronary arteries*). Plaque is made up of calcium, protein, and fatty substances. These deposits of plaque can partly clog and narrow the coronary arteries without producing any symptoms or warning signs. This puts a person at risk for a heart attack.

This test is recommended for people who are at moderate risk for heart disease. The test can find plaque deposits before symptoms develop.

## Tell a health care provider about:

- Any allergies you have.
- All medicines you are taking, including vitamins, herbs, eye drops, creams, and over-the-counter medicines.
- Any problems you or family members have had with anesthetic medicines.
- Any blood disorders you have.
- Any surgeries you have had.
- Any medical conditions you have.
- Whether you are pregnant or may be pregnant.

## What are the risks?

Generally, this is a safe procedure. However, problems may occur, including:

- Harm to a pregnant woman and her unborn baby. This test involves the use of radiation. Radiation exposure can be dangerous to a pregnant woman and her unborn baby. If you are pregnant or think you may be pregnant, you should not have this procedure done.

- Slight increase in the risk of cancer. This is because of the radiation involved in the test.

## What happens before the procedure?

Ask your health care provider for any specific instructions on how to prepare for this procedure. You may be asked to avoid products that contain caffeine, tobacco, or nicotine for 4 hours before the procedure.

## What happens during the procedure?

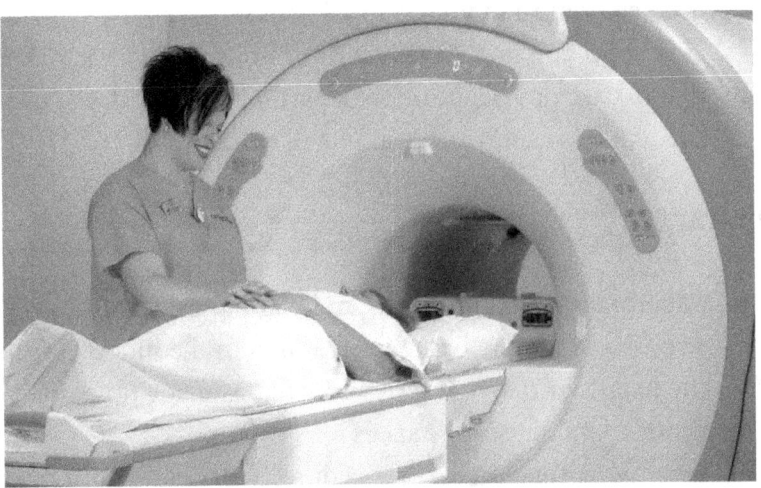

- You will undress and remove any jewelry from your neck or chest.
- You will put on a hospital gown.
- Sticky electrodes will be placed on your chest. The electrodes will be connected to an electrocardiogram (ECG) machine to record a tracing of the electrical activity of your heart.
- You will lie down on a curved bed that is attached to the CT scanner.

- You may be given medicine to slow down your heart rate so that clear pictures can be created.
- You will be moved into the CT scanner, and the CT scanner will take pictures of your heart. During this time, you will be asked to lie still and hold your breath for 2–3 seconds at a time while each picture of your heart is being taken.

The procedure may vary among health care providers and hospitals.

## What happens after the procedure?

- You can get dressed.
- You can return to your normal activities.
- It is up to you to get the results of your procedure. Ask your health care provider, or the department that is doing the procedure, when your results will be ready.

## Summary

- A coronary calcium scan is an imaging test used to look for deposits of plaque in the inner lining of the blood vessels of the heart (*coronary arteries*). Plaque is made up of calcium, protein, and fatty substances.
- Generally, this is a safe procedure. Tell your health care provider if you are pregnant or may be pregnant.
- Ask your health care provider for any specific instructions on how to prepare for this procedure.
- A CT scanner will take pictures of your heart.
- You can return to your normal activities after the scan is done.

This information is not intended to replace advice given to you by your health care provider. Make sure you discuss any questions you have with your health care provider.

# Coronary Angioplasty

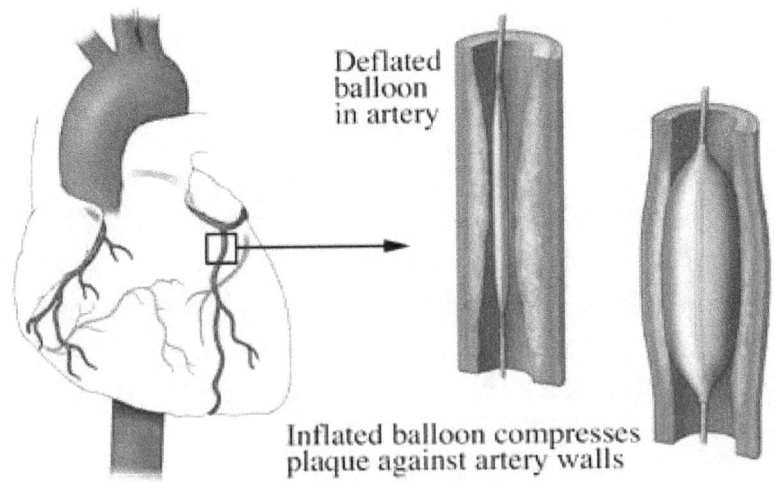

Deflated balloon in artery

Inflated balloon compresses plaque against artery walls

Coronary angioplasty is a procedure to widen a narrowed or blocked blood vessel of the heart (*coronary artery*). The artery is usually blocked by cholesterol buildup (*plaques*) in the lining of the artery walls. When a vessel in the heart becomes partially blocked, there is decreased blood flow to that area. This may lead to chest pain or a heart attack (*myocardial infarction*).

## Tell a health care provider about:

- Any allergies you have, including allergies to shellfish or contrast dye.
- All medicines you are taking, including vitamins, herbs, eye drops, creams, and over-the-counter medicines.
- Any problems you or family members have had with anesthetic medicines.
- Any blood disorders you have.
- Any surgeries you have had.
- Any medical conditions you have.

- Whether you are pregnant or may be pregnant.

## What are the risks?

Generally, this is a safe procedure. However, problems may occur, including:

- Damage to other structures or organs. This may include damage to blood vessels, leading to rupture or bleeding.
- Infection, bleeding, or bruising at the site where a small, thin tube (*catheter*) will be inserted.
- Allergic reaction to the dye or contrast that is used.
- Kidney damage from the dye or contrast that is used.
- Blood clots that can lead to a stroke or heart attack.
- Bleeding into the abdomen (*retroperitoneal bleeding*).

## What happens before the procedure?

### Staying hydrated

Follow instructions from your health care provider about hydration, which may include:

- Up to 2 hours before the procedure – you may continue to drink clear liquids, such as water, clear fruit juice, black coffee, and plain tea.

### Eating and drinking restrictions

Follow instructions from your health care provider about eating and drinking, which may include:

- 8 hours before the procedure – stop eating heavy meals or foods such as meat, fried foods, or fatty foods.
- 6 hours before the procedure – stop eating light meals or foods, such as toast or cereal.
- 2 hours before the procedure – stop drinking clear liquids.

**Medicines**

- Ask your health care provider about:

  - Changing or stopping your regular medicines. This is especially important if you are taking diabetes medicines or blood thinners.
  - Whether aspirin is recommended before this procedure.

- Ask your health care provider if you can take a sip of water with any approved medicines the morning of the procedure.

## General instructions

- Plan to have someone take you home from the hospital or clinic.
- If you will be going home right after the procedure, plan to have someone with you for 24 hours.

## What happens during the procedure?

- To reduce your risk of infection:

  - Your health care team will wash or sanitize their hands.
  - A germ-killing solution (*antiseptic*) will be used to wash the area where the catheter will be inserted. Hair may be removed from this area. The catheter may be inserted in:

    - Your groin area. This is the most common area.
    - The fold of your arm, near your elbow.
    - Your wrist.

- An IV tube will be inserted into one of your veins.
- You will be given a medicine to help you relax (*sedative*).
- You will be given a medicine to numb the area where the catheter will be inserted (*local anesthetic*).

- The catheter will be inserted into an artery.
- The catheter will be guided to the narrowed or blocked artery using a type of X-ray (*fluoroscopy*).
- When the catheter is near the heart, dye will be injected that makes the narrowing or blockage visible on the X-ray.
- Once the catheter is positioned at the narrowed or blocked portion of the blood vessel, a balloon will be inflated to make the artery wider. Expanding the balloon will crush the plaques into the wall of the vessel and improve the blood flow.
- The artery may be made wider by removing plaques using a drill, laser, or other tools.
- When the blood flow is better, the balloon will be deflated and the catheter will be removed.
- A stent may be placed. This is common in this procedure.
- After the catheter is removed, a special dressing will be placed over the insertion site.

## What happens after the procedure?

- You will need to keep the area still for a few hours, or as long as directed by your health care provider. If the procedure was done in the groin, you will be instructed not to bend or cross your legs.
- The insertion site will be checked often.
- The pulse in your feet or wrist will be checked often.
- Additional blood tests, X-rays, and an electrocardiogram (ECG) may be done.
- **Do not** drive for 24 hours if you were given a sedative.

This information is not intended to replace advice given to you by your health care provider. Make sure you discuss any questions you have with your health care provider.

# Coronary Angioplasty, Care After

This sheet gives you information about how to care for yourself after your procedure. Your health care provider may also give you more specific instructions. If you have problems or questions, contact your health care provider.

## What can I expect after the procedure?

After your procedure, it is common to have:

- Bruising at the catheter insertion site. This usually fades within 1–2 weeks.
- Blood collecting in the tissue (*hematoma*) that may be painful to the touch. It should become smaller and less tender within 1–2 weeks.

## Follow these instructions at home:

### Medicines

- Take over-the-counter and prescription medicines only as told by your health care provider.
- Blood thinners may be prescribed after your procedure to improve blood flow.

### Bathing

- You may shower 24–48 hours after the procedure or as told by your health care provider.
- **Do not** take baths, swim, or use a hot tub until your health care provider approves.

## Insertion site care

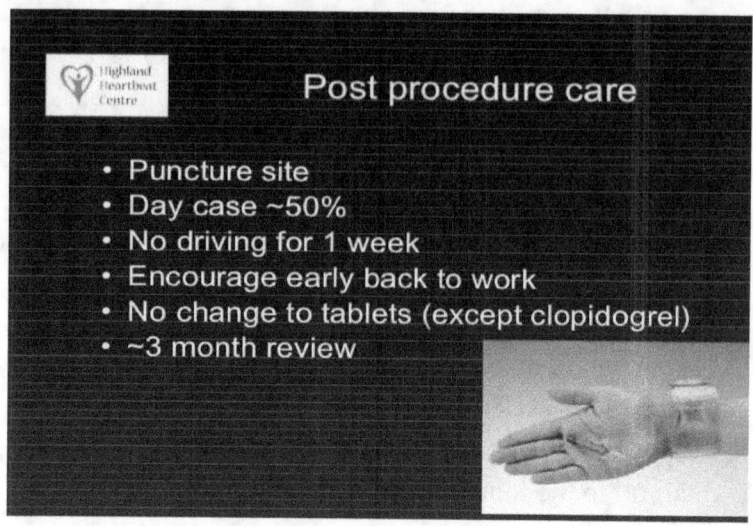

- Follow instructions from your health care provider about how to take care of your insertion site. Make sure you:
  - ➢ Wash your hands with soap and water before you change your bandage (*dressing*). If soap and water are not available, use hand sanitizer.
  - ➢ Change your dressing as told by your health care provider.
  - ➢ Gently wash the site with plain soap and water.
  - ➢ Use a clean towel to pat the area dry.
  - ➢ **Do not** rub the site, because this may cause bleeding.
  - ➢ **Do not** apply powder or lotion to the site.
- Check your insertion site every day for signs of infection. Check for:
  - ➢ More redness, swelling, or pain.
  - ➢ More fluid or blood.
  - ➢ Warmth.
  - ➢ Pus or a bad smell.

## Lifestyle

- Make any lifestyle changes as recommended by your health care provider. This may include:

  - Not using any products that contain nicotine or tobacco, such as cigarettes and e-cigarettes. If you need help quitting, ask your health care provider.
  - Managing your weight.
  - Getting regular exercise.
  - Managing your blood pressure.
  - Limiting your alcohol intake.
  - Managing other health problems, such as diabetes.

- Eat a heart-healthy diet. This should include plenty of fresh fruits and vegetables. Avoid foods that are:

  - High in salt (*sodium*).
  - Canned or highly processed.
  - High in saturated fat or sugar.
  - Fried.

## General instructions

- **Do not** lift over 10 lb (4.5 kg) for 5 days after your procedure or as told by your health care provider.
- Ask your health care provider when it is okay to:

  - Return to work or school.
  - Resume usual physical activities or sports.
  - Resume sexual activity.

- Keep all follow-up visits as told by your health care provider. This is important.

## Contact a health care provider if:

- You have a fever.
- You have chills.
- You have increased bleeding from the insertion site. Hold pressure on the site.

## Get help right away if:

- You develop chest pain or shortness of breath, feel faint, or pass out.
- You have unusual pain at the insertion site.
- You have redness, warmth, or swelling at the insertion site.
- You have drainage (other than a small amount of blood on the dressing) from the insertion site.
- The insertion site is bleeding, and the bleeding does not stop after 30 minutes of holding steady pressure on the site.
- You develop bleeding from any other place, such as from the rectum. There may be bright red blood in your urine or stool, or it may appear as black, tarry stool.

This information is not intended to replace advice given to you by your health care provider. Make sure you discuss any questions you have with your health care provider.

## Coronary Angioplasty, Care After

This sheet gives you information about how to care for yourself after your procedure. Your health care provider may also give you more specific instructions. If you have problems or questions, contact your health care provider.

# What can I expect after the procedure?

After your procedure, it is common to have:

- Bruising at the catheter insertion site. This usually fades within 1–2 weeks.
- Blood collecting in the tissue (*hematoma*) that may be painful to the touch. It should become smaller and less tender within 1–2 weeks.

## Follow these instructions at home:

### Medicines

- Take over-the-counter and prescription medicines only as told by your health care provider.
- Blood thinners may be prescribed after your procedure to improve blood flow.

### Bathing

- You may shower 24–48 hours after the procedure or as told by your health care provider.
- **Do not** take baths, swim, or use a hot tub until your health care provider approves.

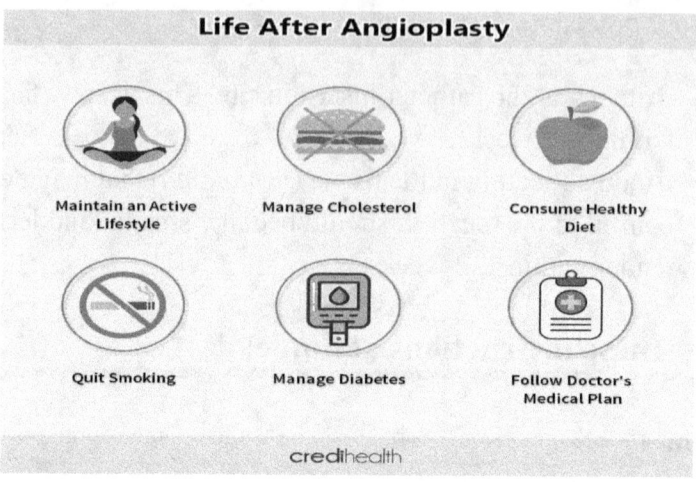

- Follow instructions from your health care provider about how to take care of your insertion site. Make sure you:

  ➢ Wash your hands with soap and water before you change your bandage (*dressing*). If soap and water are not available, use hand sanitizer.
  ➢ Change your dressing as told by your health care provider.
  ➢ Gently wash the site with plain soap and water.
  ➢ Use a clean towel to pat the area dry.
  ➢ **Do not** rub the site, because this may cause bleeding.
  ➢ **Do not** apply powder or lotion to the site.

- Check your insertion site every day for signs of infection. Check for:

  ➢ More redness, swelling, or pain.
  ➢ More fluid or blood.
  ➢ Warmth.
  ➢ Pus or a bad smell.

**Lifestyle**

- Make any lifestyle changes as recommended by your health care provider. This may include:

  - Not using any products that contain nicotine or tobacco, such as cigarettes and e-cigarettes. If you need help quitting, ask your health care provider.
  - Managing your weight.
  - Getting regular exercise.
  - Managing your blood pressure.
  - Limiting your alcohol intake.
  - Managing other health problems, such as diabetes.

- Eat a heart-healthy diet. This should include plenty of fresh fruits and vegetables. Avoid foods that are:

  - High in salt (*sodium*).
  - Canned or highly processed.
  - High in saturated fat or sugar.
  - Fried.

## General instructions

- **Do not** lift over 10 lb (4.5 kg) for 5 days after your procedure or as told by your health care provider.
- Ask your health care provider when it is okay to:

  - Return to work or school.
  - Resume usual physical activities or sports.
  - Resume sexual activity.

- Keep all follow-up visits as told by your health care provider. This is important.

## Contact a health care provider if:

- You have a fever.
- You have chills.
- You have increased bleeding from the insertion site. Hold pressure on the site.

## Get help right away if:

- You develop chest pain or shortness of breath, feel faint, or pass out.
- You have unusual pain at the insertion site.
- You have redness, warmth, or swelling at the insertion site.
- You have drainage (other than a small amount of blood on the dressing) from the insertion site.
- The insertion site is bleeding, and the bleeding does not stop after 30 minutes of holding steady pressure on the site.
- You develop bleeding from any other place, such as from the rectum. There may be bright red blood in your urine or stool, or it may appear as black, tarry stool.

This information is not intended to replace advice given to you by your health care provider. Make sure you discuss any questions you have with your health care provider.

Document Revised: 11/30/2018 Document Reviewed: 07/23/2017
Elsevier Patient Education © 2020 Elsevier Inc.

## Coronary Angiogram

A coronary angiogram is an X-ray procedure that is used to examine the arteries in the heart. Contrast dye is injected through a long, thin tube (*catheter*) into these arteries. Then X-rays are taken to show any blockage in these arteries.

You may have this procedure if you:

- Are having chest pain, or other symptoms of angina, and you are at risk for heart disease.
- Have an abnormal stress test or test of your heart's electrical activity (*electrocardiogram*, or ECG).
- Have chest pain and heart failure.
- Are having irregular heart rhythms.

A coronary angiogram or heart catheterization can show if you have valve disease or a disease of the aorta. This procedure can also be used to check the overall function of your heart muscle.

Let your health care provider know about:

- Any allergies you have, including allergies to medicines or contrast dye.
- All medicines you are taking, including vitamins, herbs, eye drops, creams, and over-the-counter medicines.
- Any problems you or family members have had with anesthetic medicines.
- Any blood disorders you have.
- Any surgeries you have had.
- Any history of kidney problems or kidney failure.
- Any medical conditions you have.
- Whether you are pregnant or may be pregnant.
- Whether you are breastfeeding.

## What are the risks?

Generally, this is a safe procedure. However, problems may occur, including:

- Infection.
- Allergic reaction to medicines or dyes that are used.
- Bleeding from the insertion site or other places.

- Damage to nearby structures, such as blood vessels, or damage to kidneys from contrast dye.
- Irregular heart rhythms.
- Stroke (rare).
- Heart attack (rare).

# What happens before the procedure?

## Staying hydrated

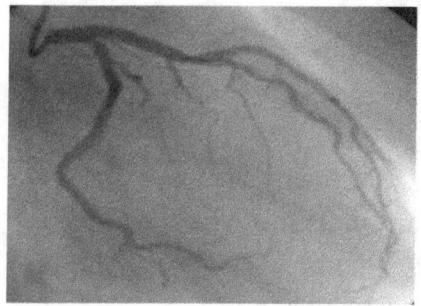

Normal coronary arteries on the left side of the heart

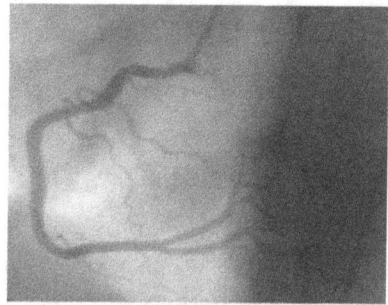

Normal coronary arteries on the right side of the heart

Follow instructions from your health care provider about hydration, which may include:

- Up to 2 hours before the procedure – you may continue to drink clear liquids, such as water, clear fruit juice, black coffee, and plain tea.

## Eating and drinking restrictions

Follow instructions from your health care provider about eating and drinking, which may include:

- 8 hours before the procedure – stop eating heavy meals or foods, such as meat, fried foods, or fatty foods.
- 6 hours before the procedure – stop eating light meals or foods, such as toast or cereal.
- 6 hours before the procedure – stop drinking milk or drinks that contain milk.
- 2 hours before the procedure – stop drinking clear liquids.

## Medicines

Ask your health care provider about:

- Changing or stopping your regular medicines. This is especially important if you are taking diabetes medicines or blood thinners.
- Taking medicines such as aspirin and ibuprofen. These medicines can thin your blood. **Do not** take these medicines unless your health care provider tells you to take them. Aspirin may be recommended before coronary angiograms even if you do not normally take it.
- Taking over-the-counter medicines, vitamins, herbs, and supplements.

## General instructions

- **Do not** use any products that contain nicotine or tobacco for at least 4 weeks before the procedure. These products include cigarettes, e-cigarettes, and chewing tobacco. If you need help quitting, ask your health care provider.
- You may have an exam or testing.
- Plan to have someone take you home from the hospital or clinic.
- If you will be going home right after the procedure, plan to have someone with you for 24 hours.
- Ask your health care provider:

➢ How your insertion site will be marked.
➢ What steps will be taken to help prevent infection. These may include:

    ○ Removing hair at the insertion site.
    ○ Washing skin with a germ-killing soap.
    ○ Taking antibiotic medicine.

## What happens during the procedure?

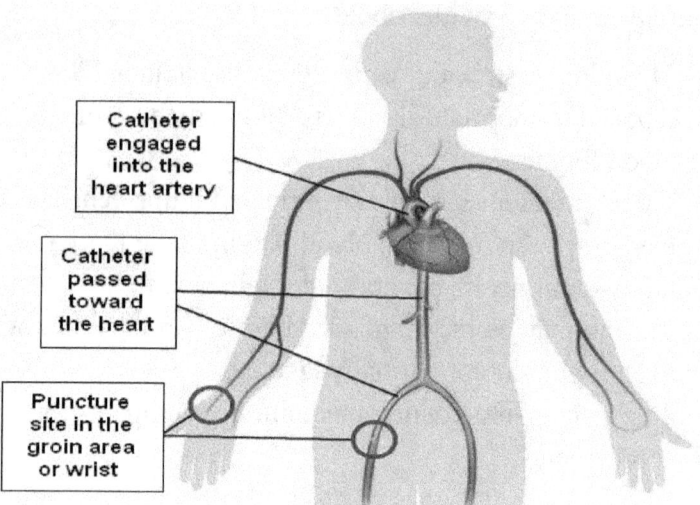

- You will lie on your back on an X-ray table.
- An IV will be inserted into one of your veins.
- Electrodes will be placed on your chest.
- You will be given one or more of the following:

➢ A medicine to help you relax (*sedative*).
➢ A medicine to numb the catheter insertion area (*local anesthetic*).

- You will be connected to a continuous ECG monitor.
- The catheter will be inserted into an artery in one of these areas:

- Your groin area in your upper thigh.
- Your wrist.
- The fold of your arm, near your elbow.

- An X-ray procedure (*fluoroscopy*) will be used to help guide the catheter to the opening of the blood vessel to be used.
- A dye will be injected into the catheter and X-rays will be taken. The dye will help to show any narrowing or blockages in the heart arteries.
- Tell your health care provider if you have chest pain or trouble breathing.
- If blockages are found, another procedure may be done to open the artery.
- The catheter will be removed after the fluoroscopy is complete.
- A bandage (*dressing*) will be placed over the insertion site. Pressure will be applied to stop bleeding.
- The IV will be removed.

The procedure may vary among health care providers and hospitals.

## What happens after the procedure?

- Your blood pressure, heart rate, breathing rate, and blood oxygen level will be monitored until you leave the hospital or clinic.
- You will need to lie still for a few hours, or for as long as told by your health care provider.

  ➤ If the procedure is done through the groin, you will be told not to bend or cross your legs.

- The insertion site and the pulse in your foot or wrist will be checked often.
- More blood tests, X-rays, and an ECG may be done.

- **Do not** drive for 24 hours if you were given a sedative during your procedure.

## Summary

- A coronary angiogram is an X-ray procedure that is used to examine the arteries in the heart.
- Contrast dye is injected through a long, thin tube (*catheter*) into each artery.
- Tell your health care provider about any allergies you have, including allergies to contrast dye.
- After the procedure, you will need to lie still for a few hours and drink plenty of fluids.

This information is not intended to replace advice given to you by your health care provider. Make sure you discuss any questions you have with your health care provider.

## Coronary Angiogram With Stent, Care After

This sheet gives you information about how to care for yourself after your procedure. Your health care provider may also give you more specific instructions. If you have problems or questions, contact your health care provider.

## What can I expect after the procedure?

After the procedure, it is common to have:

- Bruising and tenderness at the insertion site. This usually fades within 1–2 weeks.
- A collection of blood under the skin (*hematoma*). This usually decreases within 1–2 weeks.

# Follow these instructions at home:

## Medicines

- Take over-the-counter and prescription medicines only as told by your health care provider.
- If you were prescribed an antibiotic medicine, take it as told by your health care provider. **Do not** stop using the antibiotic even if you start to feel better.
- If you take medicines for diabetes, your health care provider may need to change how much you take. Ask your health care provider for specific directions about taking your diabetes medicines.
- If you are taking blood thinners:

  - Talk with your health care provider before you take any medicines that contain aspirin or NSAIDs, such as ibuprofen. These medicines increase your risk for dangerous bleeding.
  - Take your medicine exactly as told, at the same time every day.
  - Avoid activities that could cause injury or bruising, and follow instructions about how to prevent falls.
  - Wear a medical alert bracelet or carry a card that lists what medicines you take.

## Eating and drinking

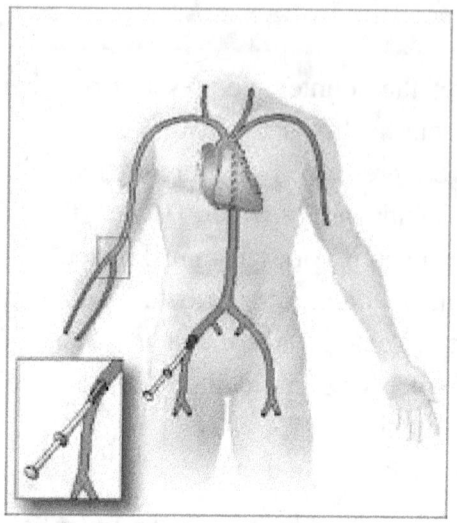

- Follow instructions from your health care provider about eating or drinking restrictions.
- Eat a heart-healthy diet that includes plenty of fresh fruits and vegetables.
- Avoid foods that are high in salt, sugar, or saturated fat. Avoid fried foods or canned or highly processed food.
- Drink enough fluid to keep your urine pale yellow.

## Alcohol use

- **Do not** drink alcohol if:
  - ➤ Your health care provider tells you not to.
  - ➤ You are pregnant, may be pregnant, or plan to become pregnant.
- If you drink alcohol:
  - ➤ Limit how much you use to:
    - ○ 0–1 drink a day for women.

o 0–2 drinks a day for men.

➤ Be aware of how much alcohol is in your drink. In the U.S., one drink equals one 12 oz bottle of beer (355 mL), one 5 oz glass of wine (148 mL), or one 1½ oz glass of hard liquor (44 mL).

## Bathing

- **Do not** take baths, swim, or use a hot tub until your health care provider approves. Ask your health care provider if you may take showers. You may only be allowed to take sponge baths.
- Gently wash the insertion site with plain soap and water.
- Pat the area dry with a clean towel. **Do not** rub. This may cause bleeding.

## Incision care

- Follow instructions from your health care provider about how to take care of your insertion area. Make sure you:

  ➤ Wash your hands with soap and water before and after you change your bandage (*dressing*). If soap and water are not available, use hand sanitizer.
  ➤ Change your dressing as told by your health care provider.
  ➤ Leave stitches (*sutures*) or adhesive strips in place. These skin closures may need to stay in place for 2 weeks or longer. If adhesive strip edges start to loosen and curl up, you may trim the loose edges. **Do not** remove adhesive strips completely unless your health care provider tells you to do that.

- **Do not** apply powder or lotion on the insertion area.
- Check your insertion area every day for signs of infection. Check for:

- ➢ Redness, swelling, or pain.
- ➢ Fluid or blood.
- ➢ Warmth.
- ➢ Pus or a bad smell.

## Activity

- **Do not** drive for 24 hours if you were given a sedative during your procedure.
- Rest as told by your health care provider.
  - ➢ Avoid sitting for a long time without moving. Get up to take short walks every 1–2 hours. This is important to improve blood flow and breathing. Ask for help if you feel weak or unsteady.
- **Do not** lift anything that is heavier than 10 lb (4.5 kg), or the limit that you are told, until your health care provider says that it is safe.
- Return to your normal activities as told by your health care provider. Ask your health care provider what activities are safe for you.

## Lifestyle

- **Do not** use any products that contain nicotine or tobacco, such as cigarettes, e-cigarettes, and chewing tobacco. If you need help quitting, ask your health care provider.
- If needed, work with your health care provider to treat other problems, such as being overweight, or having high blood pressure or diabetes.
- Get regular exercise. Do exercises as told by your health care provider.

# General instructions

- Tell all your health care providers that you have a stent. This is especially important if you are going to get imaging studies, such as MRI.
- Wear compression stockings as told by your health care provider. These stockings help to prevent blood clots and reduce swelling in your legs.
- **Do not** strain during a bowel movement if the procedure was done through your leg. Straining may cause bleeding from the insertion site.
- Keep all follow-up visits as directed by your health care provider. This is important.

## Contact a health care provider if you:

- Have a fever.
- Have chills.
- Have redness, swelling, or pain around your insertion area.
- Have fluid or blood (other than a little blood on the dressing) coming from your insertion area.
- Notice that your insertion area feels warm to the touch.
- Have pus or a bad smell coming from your insertion area.
- Have more bleeding from the insertion area. Hold pressure on the area.

# Get help right away if:

- You develop chest pain or shortness of breath.
- You feel like fainting or you faint.
- Your leg or arm becomes cool, numb, or tingly.
- You have unusual pain.
- Your insertion area is bleeding, and bleeding continues after 30 minutes of steadily held pressure.

- You develop bleeding anywhere else, including from your rectum. There may be bright red blood in your urine or stool, or you may have black, tarry stool.

**These symptoms may represent a serious problem that is an emergency. Do not wait to see if the symptoms will go away. Get medical help right away. Call your local emergency services (911 in the U.S.). Do not drive yourself to the hospital.**

## Summary

- After this procedure, it is common to have bruising and tenderness around the catheter insertion site. This will go away in a few weeks.
- Follow your health care provider's instructions about caring for your insertion site. Change dressing and clean the area as instructed.
- Eat a heart-healthy diet. Limit alcohol use. **Do not** use tobacco or nicotine.
- Contact a health care provider if you have fever or chills, or if you have pus or a bad smell coming from the site.
- Get help right away if you develop chest pain, you faint, or have bleeding at the insertion site.

This information is not intended to replace advice given to you by your health care provider. Make sure you discuss any questions you have with your health care provider.

Document Revised: 07/08/2020 Document Reviewed: 07/08/2020 Elsevier Patient Education © 2020 Elsevier Inc.

Coronary angiogram with stent placement is a procedure to widen or open a narrow blood vessel of the heart (*coronary artery*). Arteries may become blocked by cholesterol buildup (*plaques*) in the lining of the artery wall. When a coronary artery becomes partially blocked, blood flow to that area decreases. This may lead to chest pain or a heart attack (*myocardial infarction*).

A stent is a small piece of metal that looks like mesh or spring. Stent placement may be done as treatment after a heart attack, or to prevent a heart attack if a blocked artery is found by a coronary angiogram.

## Let your health care provider know about:

- Any allergies you have, including allergies to medicines or contrast dye.
- All medicines you are taking, including vitamins, herbs, eye drops, creams, and over-the-counter medicines.
- Any problems you or family members have had with anesthetic medicines.
- Any blood disorders you have.
- Any surgeries you have had.
- Any medical conditions you have, including kidney problems or kidney failure.
- Whether you are pregnant or may be pregnant.
- Whether you are breastfeeding.

## What are the risks?

Generally, this is a safe procedure. However, serious problems may occur, including:

- Damage to nearby structures or organs, such as the heart, blood vessels, or kidneys.
- A return of blockage.
- Bleeding, infection, or bruising at the insertion site.
- A collection of blood under the skin (*hematoma*) at the insertion site.
- A blood clot in another part of the body.

99

- Allergic reaction to medicines or dyes.
- Bleeding into the abdomen (*retroperitoneal bleeding*).
- Stroke (rare).
- Heart attack (rare).

# What happens before the procedure?

## Staying hydrated

Follow instructions from your health care provider about hydration, which may include:

- Up to 2 hours before the procedure – you may continue to drink clear liquids, such as water, clear fruit juice, black coffee, and plain tea.

## Eating and drinking restrictions

Follow instructions from your health care provider about eating and drinking, which may include:

- 8 hours before the procedure – stop eating heavy meals or foods, such as meat, fried foods, or fatty foods.
- 6 hours before the procedure – stop eating light meals or foods, such as toast or cereal.
- 2 hours before the procedure – stop drinking clear liquids.

## Medicines

Ask your health care provider about:

- Changing or stopping your regular medicines. This is especially important if you are taking diabetes medicines or blood thinners.
- Taking medicines such as aspirin and ibuprofen. These medicines can thin your blood. **Do not** take these medicines unless your health care provider tells you to take them.

- Generally, aspirin is recommended before a thin tube, called a catheter, is passed through a blood vessel and inserted into the heart (*cardiac catheterization*).
- Taking over-the-counter medicines, vitamins, herbs, and supplements.

## General instructions

- **Do not** use any products that contain nicotine or tobacco for at least 4 weeks before the procedure. These products include cigarettes, e-cigarettes, and chewing tobacco. If you need help quitting, ask your health care provider.
- Plan to have someone take you home from the hospital or clinic.
- If you will be going home right after the procedure, plan to have someone with you for 24 hours.
- You may have tests and imaging procedures.
- Ask your health care provider:
  - How your insertion site will be marked. Ask which artery will be used for the procedure.
  - What steps will be taken to help prevent infection. These may include:
    - Removing hair at the insertion site.
    - Washing skin with a germ-killing soap.
    - Taking antibiotic medicine.

# What happens during the procedure?

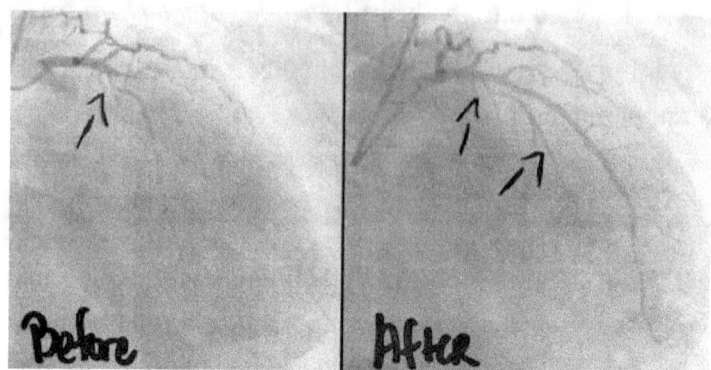

shutterstock.com • 137026661

- An IV will be inserted into one of your veins.
- Electrodes may be placed on your chest to monitor your heart rate during the procedure.
- You will be given one or more of the following:
  - ➤ A medicine to help you relax (*sedative*).
  - ➤ A medicine to numb the area (*local anesthetic*) for catheter insertion.
- A small incision will be made for catheter insertion.
- The catheter will be inserted into an artery using a guide wire. The location may be in your groin, your wrist, or the fold of your arm (near your elbow).
- An X-ray procedure (*fluoroscopy*) will be used to help guide the catheter to the opening of the heart arteries.
- A dye will be injected into the catheter. X-rays will be taken. The dye helps to show where any narrowing or blockages are located in the arteries.
- Tell your health care provider if you have chest pain or trouble breathing.
- A tiny wire will be guided to the blocked spot, and a balloon will be inflated to make the artery wider.

102

- The stent will be expanded to crush the plaques into the wall of the vessel. The stent will hold the area open and improve the blood flow. Most stents have a drug coating to reduce the risk of the stent narrowing over time.
- The artery may be made wider using a drill, laser, or other tools that remove plaques.
- The catheter will be removed when the blood flow improves. The stent will stay where it was placed, and the lining of the artery will grow over it.
- A bandage (*dressing*) will be placed on the insertion site. Pressure will be applied to stop bleeding.
- The IV will be removed.

This procedure may vary among health care providers and hospitals.

## What happens after the procedure?

- Your blood pressure, heart rate, breathing rate, and blood oxygen level will be monitored until you leave the hospital or clinic.
- If the procedure is done through the leg, you will lie flat in bed for a few hours or for as long as told by your health care provider. You will be instructed not to bend or cross your legs.
- The insertion site and the pulse in your foot or wrist will be checked often.
- You may have more blood tests, X-rays, and a test that records the electrical activity of your heart (*electrocardiogram*, or ECG).
- **Do not** drive for 24 hours if you were given a sedative during your procedure.

# Summary

- Coronary angiogram with stent placement is a procedure to widen or open a narrowed coronary artery. This is done to treat heart problems.
- Before the procedure, let your health care provider know about all the medical conditions and surgeries you have or have had.
- This is a safe procedure. However, some problems may occur, including damage to nearby structures or organs, bleeding, blood clots, or allergies.
- Follow your health care provider's instructions about eating, drinking, medicines, and other lifestyle changes, such as quitting tobacco use before the procedure.

This information is not intended to replace advice given to you by your health care provider. Make sure you discuss any questions you have with your health care provider.

# Coronary Artery Bypass Grafting

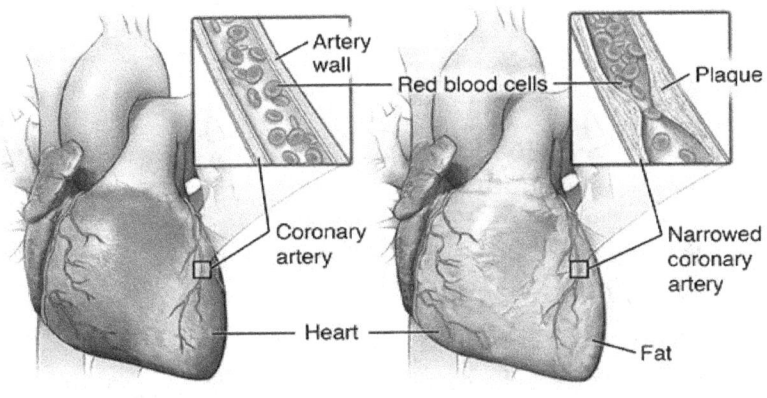

**Normal heart and artery**    **Artery with plaque buildup**

Coronary artery bypass grafting (CABG) is a surgery that is done when arteries of the heart have become narrow or blocked. This is often caused by the buildup of fat called plaques. These arteries give the heart the oxygen and nutrients it needs to pump blood to your body.

During CABG, a section of blood vessel from another part of the body is taken. This section is called a graft. The graft is placed where there is narrowing or blockage.

## Tell your doctor about:

- Any allergies you have.
- All medicines you are taking. Tell him or her about any steroids, blood thinners, vitamins, herbs, eye drops, creams, and over-the-counter medicines.
- Any problems you or family members have had with anesthetic medicines.
- Any blood disorders you have.

- Any surgeries you have had.
- Any medical conditions you have.
- Whether you are pregnant or may be pregnant.

## What are the risks?

Generally, this is a safe procedure. However, problems may occur, including:

- Bleeding. You may need to get blood through an IV tube (*transfusions*).
- Infection.
- Allergic reactions to medicines or dyes.
- Pain at the surgical site.
- Damage to organs or other parts of the body.
- Short-term memory loss, confusion, and personality changes.
- Heart rhythm problems (*arrhythmias*).
- Stroke.
- Heart attack during or after surgery.
- Kidney failure.

## What happens before the procedure?

### Staying hydrated

Follow instructions from your doctor about hydration. These may include:

- Up to 2 hours before the procedure – you may continue to drink clear liquids, such as:
  - Water.
  - Clear fruit juice.
  - Black coffee.
  - Plain tea.

## Eating and drinking

Follow instructions from your doctor about eating and drinking. These may include:

- 8 hours before the procedure – stop eating heavy meals or foods, such as:
  - ➢ Meat.
  - ➢ Fried foods.
  - ➢ Fatty foods.
- 6 hours before the procedure – stop eating light meals or foods, such as:
  - ➢ Toast.
  - ➢ Cereal.
- 6 hours before the procedure – stop drinking milk or drinks that contain milk.
- 2 hours before the procedure – stop drinking clear liquids.

## Medicines

- Take over-the-counter and prescription medicines only as told by your doctor.
- Ask your doctor about:
  - ➢ Changing or stopping your normal medicines. This is important.
  - ➢ Taking aspirin and ibuprofen. **Do not** take these medicines unless your doctor tells you to take them.
  - ➢ Taking over-the-counter medicines, vitamins, herbs, and supplements.

## General instructions

- Ask your doctor:

- ➤ How your surgery site will be marked.
- ➤ What steps will be taken to help prevent the spread of germs. These may include:
  - ○ Removing hair at the surgery site.
  - ○ Washing skin with a germ-killing soap.
  - ○ Taking antibiotic medicine.
- You may be asked to shower with a germ-killing soap.
- For 3–6 weeks before the CABG, **do not** use any products that contain nicotine or tobacco. These include cigarettes, e-cigarettes, and chewing tobacco. Quitting smoking is one of the best things you can do for your heart health. If you need help quitting, ask your doctor.
- Talk with your doctor about where the grafts will be taken from for your surgery.

## What happens during the procedure?

- An IV tube will be placed into one of your veins.
- You will be given one or more of the following:
  - ➤ A medicine to help you relax (*sedative*).
  - ➤ A medicine to make you fall asleep (*general anesthetic*).
- A cut (*incision*) will be made down the front of the chest through the breastbone (*sternum*).
- The breastbone will be opened so your heart can be seen.
- You may or may not be placed on a heart-lung bypass machine.
  - ➤ If this machine is used, your heart will be briefly stopped.
  - ➤ This machine will give oxygen to your blood while your heart is being worked on.

- A section of blood vessel will be removed from another part of your body (often the chest, arm, or leg).
- The blood vessel will be attached above and below the blocked artery of your heart. This may be done on more than one artery of the heart.
- You will be taken off the heart-lung machine if it was used.
- If your heart was stopped, it will be restarted.
- Your chest will be closed with special wire that will hold your bones together as they heal.
- Your cuts will be closed with stitches (*sutures*), skin glue, or skin tape (*adhesive*) strips.
- A bandage (*dressing*) will be placed over the cuts.
- Tubes will stay in your chest. They will be connected to a device that will help drain fluid and reinflate the lungs.

The procedure may vary among doctors and hospitals.

## What happens after the procedure?

- You will be monitored until you leave the hospital. This includes checking your blood pressure, heart rate, breathing rate, and blood oxygen level.
- You may wake up with a tube in your throat. This tube will help you breathe. You may be connected to a breathing machine. You will not be able to talk when the tube is in. The tube will be taken out when it is safe.
- You will be groggy and may have some pain. You will be given medicine to help the pain.
- You may be in the intensive care unit for 1–2 days.
- You may be given oxygen to help you breathe.
- You will be shown how to do deep breathing exercises.
- You may have to wear compression stockings. These stockings help to prevent blood clots and reduce swelling in your legs.

- You may be given new medicines to take.
- Cardiac rehab will be started while you are in the hospital. This may include education and exercises to help you recover from your surgery.

## Summary

- During CABG, a section of blood vessel from another part of the body is taken out. It is then placed where there is narrowing or blockage.
- For 3–6 weeks before the procedure, **do not** use any products that contain nicotine or tobacco. Quitting smoking is one of the best things you can do for your heart health. If you need help quitting, ask your doctor.
- You may wake up with a tube in your throat. This tube will help you breathe. You will not be able to talk when the tube is in. The tube will be taken out when it is safe.

This information is not intended to replace advice given to you by your health care provider. Make sure you discuss any questions you have with your health car

# Coronary Artery Bypass Grafting, Care After

This sheet gives you information about how to care for yourself after your procedure. Your health care provider may also give you more specific instructions. If you have problems or questions, contact your health care provider.

## What can I expect after the procedure?

After the procedure, it is common to have:

- Nausea.
- Lack of appetite.
- Constipation.
- Weakness and fatigue.
- Depression or irritability.
- Pain or discomfort in your incision areas.

## Follow these instructions at home:

### Medicines

Take over-the-counter and prescription medicines only as told by your health care provider. **Do not** stop taking medicines or start any new medicines without approval from your health care provider.

- If you were prescribed an antibiotic medicine, take it as told by your health care provider. **Do not** stop using the antibiotic even if you start to feel better.

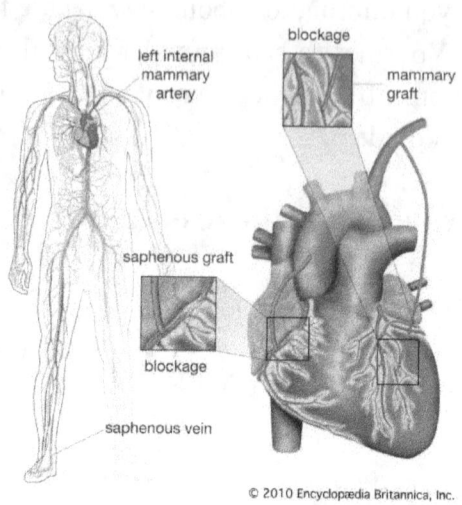

© 2010 Encyclopædia Britannica, Inc.

- Follow instructions from your health care provider about how to take care of your incisions. Make sure you:
  - ➢ Wash your hands with soap and water before and after you change your bandage (*dressing*). If soap and water are not available, use hand sanitizer.
  - ➢ Change your dressing as told by your health care provider.
  - ➢ Leave stitches (*sutures*), skin glue, or adhesive strips in place. These skin closures may need to stay in place for 2 weeks or longer. If adhesive strip edges start to loosen and curl up, you may trim the loose edges. **Do not** remove adhesive strips completely unless your health care provider tells you to do that.

- Keep incision areas clean, dry, and protected.
- Check your incision areas every day for signs of infection. Check for:
  - ➢ More redness, swelling, or pain.

112

- ➢ More fluid or blood.
- ➢ Warmth.
- ➢ Pus or a bad smell.
- If incisions were made in your legs:
  - ➢ Avoid crossing your legs.
  - ➢ Avoid sitting for long periods of time. Change positions every 30 minutes.
  - ➢ Raise (*elevate*) your legs when you are sitting.

## Bathing

- **Do not** take baths, swim, or use a hot tub until your health care provider approves.
- Only take sponge baths. Pat the incisions dry. **Do not** rub incisions with a washcloth or towel.
- Ask your health care provider when you can shower.

## Eating and drinking

### Healthy Heart Diet Chart

TOTAL CALORIES
(kcals/Day)
2730

- Eat foods that are high in fiber, such as beans, nuts, whole grains, and raw fruits and vegetables. Meats, if eaten, should be lean cut. Avoid canned, processed, and fried foods. This

113

can help prevent constipation and is a recommended part of a heart-healthy diet.

- Drink enough fluid to keep your urine pale yellow.
- **Do not** drink alcohol until your recovery is complete. Ask your health care provider when it is safe to drink alcohol.

## Activity

- Rest and limit your activity as told by your health care provider. You may be instructed to:

  ➢ Stop any activity right away if you have chest pain, shortness of breath, irregular heartbeats, or dizziness. Get help right away if you have any of these symptoms.
  
  ➢ Move around frequently for short periods or take short walks as told by your health care provider. Gradually increase your activities.
  
  ➢ Avoid lifting, pushing, or pulling anything that is heavier than 10 lb (4.5 kg) for at least 6 weeks or as told by your health care provider.

- Participate in physical therapy or a cardiac rehabilitation program as told by your health care provider.

  ➢ Physical therapy involves doing exercises to maintain movement, strengthen your muscles, and build your endurance.
  
  ➢ A cardiac rehabilitation program is a treatment program to improve your health and well-being through exercise training, education, and counseling.

- **Do not** drive until your health care provider approves.
- Ask your health care provider when you may return to work.
- Ask your health care provider when you may resume sexual activity.

# General instructions

- **Do not** drive or use heavy machinery while taking prescription pain medicine.
- **Do not** use any products that contain nicotine or tobacco, such as cigarettes, e-cigarettes, and chewing tobacco. If you need help quitting, ask your health care provider.
- Take 2–3 deep breaths every few hours during the day, while you recover. This helps expand your lungs and prevent complications like pneumonia after surgery.
- If you were given a device called an incentive spirometer, use it several times a day to practice deep breathing. Support your chest with a pillow or your arms when you take deep breaths or cough.
- Wear compression stockings as told by your health care provider. These stockings help to prevent blood clots and reduce swelling in your legs.
- Weigh yourself every day. This helps identify if your body is holding (*retaining*) fluid that may make your heart and lungs work harder.
- Keep all follow-up visits as told by your health care provider. This is important.

# Contact a health care provider if:

- You have more redness, swelling, or pain around any incision.
- You have more fluid or blood coming from any incision.
- Any incision feels warm to the touch.
- You have pus or a bad smell coming from any incision.
- You have a fever.
- You have swelling in your ankles or legs.
- You have pain in your legs.
- You gain 2 lb (0.9 kg) or more a day.

115

- You are nauseous or you vomit.
- You have diarrhea.

## Get help right away if:

- You have chest pain that spreads to your jaw or arms.
- You are short of breath.
- You have a fast or irregular heartbeat.
- You notice a "clicking" in your breastbone (*sternum*) when you move.
- You have any symptoms of a stroke. **"BE FAST"** is an easy way to remember the main warning signs of a stroke:

  - ➢ **B - Balance.** Signs are dizziness, sudden trouble walking, or loss of balance.
  - ➢ **E - Eyes.** Signs are trouble seeing or a sudden change in vision.
  - ➢ **F - Face.** Signs are sudden weakness or numbness of the face, or the face or eyelid drooping on one side.
  - ➢ **A - Arms.** Signs are weakness or numbness in an arm. This happens suddenly and usually on one side of the body.
  - ➢ **S - Speech.** Signs are sudden trouble speaking, slurred speech, or trouble understanding what people say.
  - ➢ **T - Time.** Time to call emergency services. Write down what time symptoms started.

- You have other signs of a stroke, such as:

  - ➢ A sudden, severe headache with no known cause.
  - ➢ Nausea or vomiting.
  - ➢ Seizure.

**These symptoms may represent a serious problem that is an emergency. Do not wait to see if the symptoms will go away. Get**

**medical help right away. Call your local emergency services (911 in the U.S.). Do not drive yourself to the hospital.**

## Summary

- After the procedure, it is common to have pain or discomfort in the incision areas.
- **Do not** take baths, swim, or use a hot tub until your health care provider approves.
- Gradually increase your activities. You may need physical therapy or cardiac rehabilitation to help strengthen your muscles and build your endurance.
- Weigh yourself every day. This helps identify if your body is holding (*retaining*) fluid that may make your heart and lungs work harder.

This information is not intended to replace advice given to you by your health care provider. Make sure you discuss any questions you have with your health care provider.

## Summary

- Atherosclerosis is narrowing and hardening of the arteries.
- Arteries can become narrow or clogged with a buildup of fat, cholesterol, calcium, and other substances (plaque).
- This condition may not cause any symptoms. If you do have symptoms, they are caused by damage to an area of your body that is not getting enough blood.
- Treatment may include lifestyle changes and medicines. In some cases, surgery is needed.

# Cardiac Ablation, Care After

This sheet gives you information about how to care for yourself after your procedure. Your health care provider may also give you more specific instructions. If you have problems or questions, contact your health care provider.

## What can I expect after the procedure?

After the procedure, it is common to have:

- Bruising around your puncture site.
- Tenderness around your puncture site.
- Skipped heartbeats.
- Tiredness (*fatigue*).

## Follow these instructions at home:

### Puncture site care

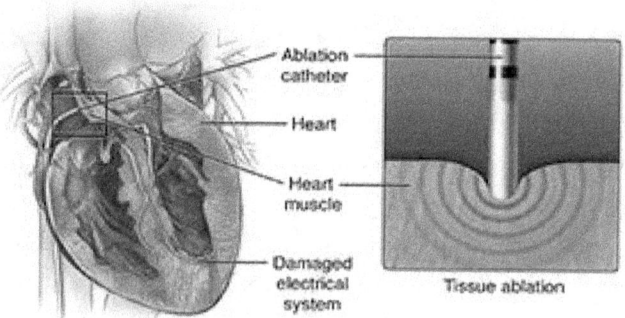

Catheter ablation

- Follow instructions from your health care provider about how to take care of your puncture site. Make sure you:

- Wash your hands with soap and water before you change your bandage (*dressing*). If soap and water are not available, use hand sanitizer.
- Change your dressing as told by your health care provider.
- Leave stitches (*sutures*), skin glue, or adhesive strips in place. These skin closures may need to stay in place for up to 2 weeks. If adhesive strip edges start to loosen and curl up, you may trim the loose edges. **Do not** remove adhesive strips completely unless your health care provider tells you to do that.

- Check your puncture site every day for signs of infection. Check for:

  - Redness, swelling, or pain.
  - Fluid or blood. If your puncture site starts to bleed, lie down on your back, apply firm pressure to the area, and contact your health care provider.
  - Warmth.
  - Pus or a bad smell.

## Driving

- Ask your health care provider when it is safe for you to drive again after the procedure.
- **Do not** drive or use heavy machinery while taking prescription pain medicine.
- **Do not** drive for 24 hours if you were given a medicine to help you relax (*sedative*) during your procedure.

## Activity

- Avoid activities that take a lot of effort for at least 3 days after your procedure.

- **Do not** lift anything that is heavier than 10 lb (4.5 kg), or the limit that you are told, until your health care provider says that it is safe.
- Return to your normal activities as told by your health care provider. Ask your health care provider what activities are safe for you.

## General instructions

- Take over-the-counter and prescription medicines only as told by your health care provider.
- **Do not** use any products that contain nicotine or tobacco, such as cigarettes and e-cigarettes. If you need help quitting, ask your health care provider.
- **Do not** take baths, swim, or use a hot tub until your health care provider approves.
- **Do not** drink alcohol for 24 hours after your procedure.
- Keep all follow-up visits as told by your health care provider. This is important.

## Contact a health care provider if:

- You have redness, mild swelling, or pain around your puncture site.
- You have fluid or blood coming from your puncture site that stops after applying firm pressure to the area.
- Your puncture site feels warm to the touch.
- You have pus or a bad smell coming from your puncture site.
- You have a fever.
- You have chest pain or discomfort that spreads to your neck, jaw, or arm.
- You are sweating a lot.
- You feel nauseous.

- You have a fast or irregular heartbeat.
- You have shortness of breath.
- You are dizzy or light-headed and feel the need to lie down.
- You have pain or numbness in the arm or leg closest to your puncture site.

## Get help right away if:

- Your puncture site suddenly swells.
- Your puncture site is bleeding and the bleeding does not stop after applying firm pressure to the area.

**These symptoms may represent a serious problem that is an emergency. Do not wait to see if the symptoms will go away. Get medical help right away. Call your local emergency services (911 in the U.S.). Do not drive yourself to the hospital.**

## Summary

- After the procedure, it is normal to have bruising and tenderness at the puncture site in your groin, neck, or forearm.
- Check your puncture site every day for signs of infection.
- Get help right away if your puncture site is bleeding and the bleeding does not stop after applying firm pressure to the area. This is a medical emergency.

This information is not intended to replace advice given to you by your health care provider. Make sure you discuss any questions you have with your health care provider.

Document Revised: 11/30/2018 Document Reviewed: 03/29/2018
Elsevier Patient Education © 2020 Elsevier Inc.

# Cardiac Ablation

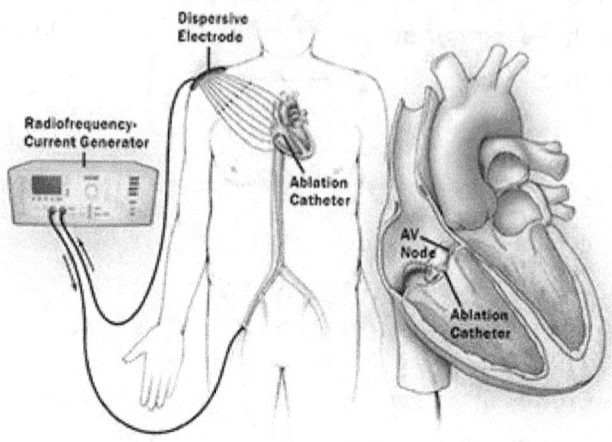

Cardiac ablation is a procedure to stop some heart tissue from causing problems. The heart has many electrical connections. Sometimes these connections make the heart beat very fast or irregularly. Removing some problem areas can improve the heart rhythm or make it normal.

## What happens before the procedure?

- Follow instructions from your doctor about what you cannot eat or drink.
- Ask your doctor about:
  - ➤ Changing or stopping your normal medicines. This is important if you take diabetes medicines or blood thinners.
  - ➤ Taking medicines such as aspirin and ibuprofen. These medicines can thin your blood. **Do not** take these medicines before your procedure if your doctor tells you not to.
- Plan to have someone take you home.

- If you will be going home right after the procedure, plan to have someone with you for 24 hours.

## What happens during the procedure?

- To lower your risk of infection:
  - ➢ Your health care team will wash or sanitize their hands.
  - ➢ Your skin will be washed with soap.
  - ➢ Hair may be removed from your neck or groin.
- An IV tube will be put into one of your veins.
- You will be given a medicine to help you relax (*sedative*).
- Skin on your neck or groin will be numbed.
- A cut (*incision*) will be made in your neck or groin.
- A needle will be put through your cut and into a vein in your neck or groin.
- A tube (*catheter*) will be put into the needle. The tube will be moved to your heart. X-rays (*fluoroscopy*) will be used to help guide the tube.
- Small devices (*electrodes*) on the tip of the tube will send out electrical currents.
- Dye may be put through the tube. This helps your surgeon see your heart.
- Electrical energy will be used to scar (*ablate*) some heart tissue. Your surgeon may use:
  - ➢ Heat (radiofrequency energy).
  - ➢ Laser energy.
  - ➢ Extreme cold (cryoablation).
- The tube will be taken out.
- Pressure will be held on your cut. This helps stop bleeding.
- A bandage (*dressing*) will be put on your cut.

The procedure may vary.

## What happens after the procedure?

- You will be monitored until your medicines have worn off.
- Your cut will be watched for bleeding. You will need to lie still for a few hours.
- **Do not** drive for 24 hours or as long as your doctor tells you.

## Summary

- Cardiac ablation is a procedure to stop some heart tissue from causing problems.
- Electrical energy will be used to scar (*ablate*) some heart tissue.

This information is not intended to replace advice given to you by your health care provider. Make sure you discuss any questions you have with your health care provider.

Document Revised: 11/30/2018 Document Reviewed: 11/06/2017
Elsevier Patient Education © 2020 Elsevier Inc.

# Cardiac Ablation

Cardiac ablation is a procedure to disable (*ablate*) a small amount of heart tissue in very specific places. The heart has many electrical connections. Sometimes these connections are abnormal and can cause the heart to beat very fast or irregularly. Ablating some of the problem areas can improve the heart rhythm or return it to normal. Ablation may be done for people who:

- Have Wolff-Parkinson-White syndrome.
- Have fast heart rhythms (*tachycardia*).
- Have taken medicines for an abnormal heart rhythm (*arrhythmia*) that were not effective or caused side effects.
- Have a high-risk heartbeat that may be life-threatening.

During the procedure, a small incision is made in the neck or the groin, and a long, thin, flexible tube (*catheter*) is inserted into the incision and moved to the heart. Small devices (*electrodes*) on the tip of the catheter will send out electrical currents. A type of X-ray (*fluoroscopy*) will be used to help guide the catheter and to provide images of the heart.

## Tell a health care provider about:

- Any allergies you have.
- All medicines you are taking, including vitamins, herbs, eye drops, creams, and over-the-counter medicines.
- Any problems you or family members have had with anesthetic medicines.
- Any blood disorders you have.
- Any surgeries you have had.
- Any medical conditions you have, such as kidney failure.
- Whether you are pregnant or may be pregnant.

# What are the risks?

Generally, this is a safe procedure. However, problems may occur, including:

- Infection.
- Bruising and bleeding at the catheter insertion site.
- Bleeding into the chest, especially into the sac that surrounds the heart. This is a serious complication.
- Stroke or blood clots.
- Damage to other structures or organs.
- Allergic reaction to medicines or dyes.
- Need for a permanent pacemaker if the normal electrical system is damaged. A pacemaker is a small computer that sends electrical signals to the heart and helps your heart beat normally.
- The procedure not being fully effective. This may not be recognized until months later. Repeat ablation procedures are sometimes required.

## What happens before the procedure?

- Follow instructions from your health care provider about eating or drinking restrictions.
- Ask your health care provider about:
  - ➢ Changing or stopping your regular medicines. This is especially important if you are taking diabetes medicines or blood thinners.
  - ➢ Taking medicines such as aspirin and ibuprofen. These medicines can thin your blood. **Do not** take these medicines before your procedure if your health care provider instructs you not to.

- Plan to have someone take you home from the hospital or clinic.
- If you will be going home right after the procedure, plan to have someone with you for 24 hours.

## What happens during the procedure?

- To lower your risk of infection:
  - ➤ Your health care team will wash or sanitize their hands.
  - ➤ Your skin will be washed with soap.
  - ➤ Hair may be removed from the incision area.
- An IV tube will be inserted into one of your veins.
- You will be given a medicine to help you relax (*sedative*).
- The skin on your neck or groin will be numbed.
- An incision will be made in your neck or your groin.
- A needle will be inserted through the incision and into a large vein in your neck or groin.
- A catheter will be inserted into the needle and moved to your heart.
- Dye may be injected through the catheter to help your surgeon see the area of the heart that needs treatment.
- Electrical currents will be sent from the catheter to ablate heart tissue in desired areas.
- There are three types of energy that may be used to ablate heart tissue:
  - ➤ Heat (radiofrequency energy).
  - ➤ Laser energy.
  - ➤ Extreme cold (cryoablation).
- When the necessary tissue has been ablated, the catheter will be removed.
- Pressure will be held on the catheter insertion area to prevent excessive bleeding.

- A bandage (*dressing*) will be placed over the catheter insertion area.

The procedure may vary among health care providers and hospitals.

## What happens after the procedure?

- Your blood pressure, heart rate, breathing rate, and blood oxygen level will be monitored until the medicines you were given have worn off.
- Your catheter insertion area will be monitored for bleeding. You will need to lie still for a few hours to ensure that you do not bleed from the catheter insertion area.
- **Do not** drive for 24 hours or as long as directed by your health care provider.

## Summary

- Cardiac ablation is a procedure to disable (*ablate*) a small amount of heart tissue in very specific places. Ablating some of the problem areas can improve the heart rhythm or return it to normal.
- During the procedure, electrical currents will be sent from the catheter to ablate heart tissue in desired areas.

This information is not intended to replace advice given to you by your health care provider. Make sure you discuss any questions you have with your health care provider.

# Cardiac Nuclear Scan

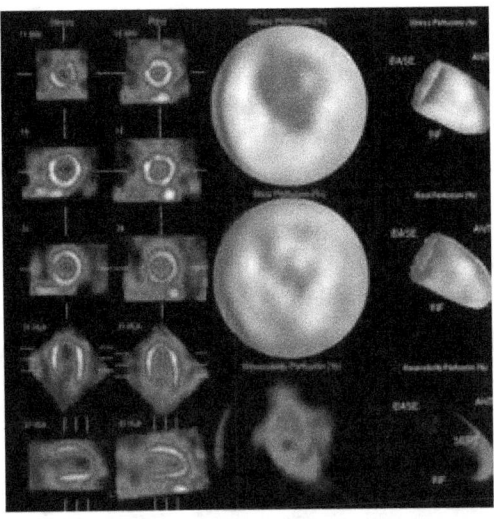

A cardiac nuclear scan is a test that measures blood flow to the heart when a person is resting and when he or she is exercising. The test looks for problems such as:

- Not enough blood reaching a portion of the heart.
- The heart muscle not working normally.

You may need this test if:

- You have heart disease.
- You have had abnormal lab results.
- You have had heart surgery or a balloon procedure to open up blocked arteries (*angioplasty*).
- You have chest pain.
- You have shortness of breath.

In this test, a radioactive dye (*tracer*) is injected into your bloodstream. After the tracer has traveled to your heart, an imaging device is used to measure how much of the tracer is absorbed by or distributed to various areas of your heart. This procedure is usually done at a hospital and takes 2–4 hours.

## Tell a health care provider about:

- Any allergies you have.
- All medicines you are taking, including vitamins, herbs, eye drops, creams, and over-the-counter medicines.
- Any problems you or family members have had with anesthetic medicines.
- Any blood disorders you have.
- Any surgeries you have had.
- Any medical conditions you have.
- Whether you are pregnant or may be pregnant.

## What are the risks?

Generally, this is a safe procedure. However, problems may occur, including:

- Serious chest pain and heart attack. This is only a risk if the stress portion of the test is done.
- Rapid heartbeat.
- Sensation of warmth in your chest. This usually passes quickly.
- Allergic reaction to the tracer.

## What happens before the procedure?

- Ask your health care provider about changing or stopping your regular medicines. This is especially important if you are taking diabetes medicines or blood thinners.
- Follow instructions from your health care provider about eating or drinking restrictions.
- Remove your jewelry on the day of the procedure.

# What happens during the procedure?

- An IV will be inserted into one of your veins.
- Your health care provider will inject a small amount of radioactive tracer through the IV.
- You will wait for 20–40 minutes while the tracer travels through your bloodstream.
- Your heart activity will be monitored with an electrocardiogram (ECG).
- You will lie down on an exam table.
- Images of your heart will be taken for about 15–20 minutes.
- You may also have a stress test. For this test, one of the following may be done:

  - You will exercise on a treadmill or stationary bike. While you exercise, your heart's activity will be monitored with an ECG, and your blood pressure will be checked.
  - You will be given medicines that will increase blood flow to parts of your heart. This is done if you are unable to exercise.

- When blood flow to your heart has peaked, a tracer will again be injected through the IV.
- After 20–40 minutes, you will get back on the exam table and have more images taken of your heart.
- Depending on the type of tracer used, scans may need to be repeated 3–4 hours later.
- Your IV line will be removed when the procedure is over.

The procedure may vary among health care providers and hospitals.

# What happens after the procedure?

- Unless your health care provider tells you otherwise, you may return to your normal schedule, including diet, activities, and medicines.
- Unless your health care provider tells you otherwise, you may increase your fluid intake. This will help to flush the contrast dye from your body. Drink enough fluid to keep your urine pale yellow.
- Ask your health care provider, or the department that is doing the test:
  - ➢ When will my results be ready?
  - ➢ How will I get my results?

## Summary

- A cardiac nuclear scan measures the blood flow to the heart when a person is resting and when he or she is exercising.
- Tell your health care provider if you are pregnant.
- Before the procedure, ask your health care provider about changing or stopping your regular medicines. This is especially important if you are taking diabetes medicines or blood thinners.
- After the procedure, unless your health care provider tells you otherwise, increase your fluid intake. This will help flush the contrast dye from your body.
- After the procedure, unless your health care provider tells you otherwise, you may return to your normal schedule, including diet, activities, and medicines.

This information is not intended to replace advice given to you by your health care provider. Make sure you discuss any questions you have with your health care provider.

# Cardiac Rehabilitation

## What is cardiac rehabilitation?

Cardiac rehabilitation is a treatment program that helps improve the health and well-being of people who have heart problems. Cardiac rehabilitation includes exercise training, education, and counseling to help you get stronger and return to an active lifestyle. This program can help you get better faster and reduce any future hospital stays.

## Why might I need cardiac rehabilitation?

Cardiac rehabilitation programs can help when you have or have had:

- A heart attack.
- Heart failure.
- Peripheral artery disease.
- Coronary artery disease.
- Angina.
- Lung or breathing problems.

Cardiac rehabilitation programs are also used when you have had:

- Coronary artery bypass graft surgery.
- Heart valve replacement.
- Heart stent placement.
- Heart transplant.
- Aneurysm repair.

## What are the benefits of cardiac rehabilitation?

Cardiac rehabilitation can help you:

- Reduce problems like chest pain and trouble breathing.

133

- Change risk factors that contribute to heart disease, such as:
- Smoking.
- High blood pressure.
- High cholesterol.
- Diabetes.
- Being inactive.
- Weighing over 30% more than your ideal weight.
- Diet.
- Improve your emotional outlook so you feel:
- More hopeful.
- Better about yourself.
- More confident about taking care of yourself.
- Get support from health experts as well as other people with similar problems.
- Learn healthy ways to manage stress.
- Learn how to manage and understand your medicines.
- Teach your family about your condition and how to participate in your recovery.

## What happens in cardiac rehabilitation?

You will be assessed by a cardiac rehabilitation team. They will check your health history and do a physical exam. You may need blood tests, exercise stress tests, and other evaluations to make sure that you are ready to start cardiac rehabilitation.

The cardiac rehabilitation team works with you to make a plan based on your health and goals. Your program will be tailored to fit you and your needs and may change as you progress. You may work with a health care team that includes:

- Doctors.
- Nurses.
- Dietitians.
- Psychologists.

- Exercise specialists.
- Physical and occupational therapists.

## What are the phases of cardiac rehabilitation?

A cardiac rehabilitation program is often divided into phases. You advance from one phase to the next.

### Phase 1

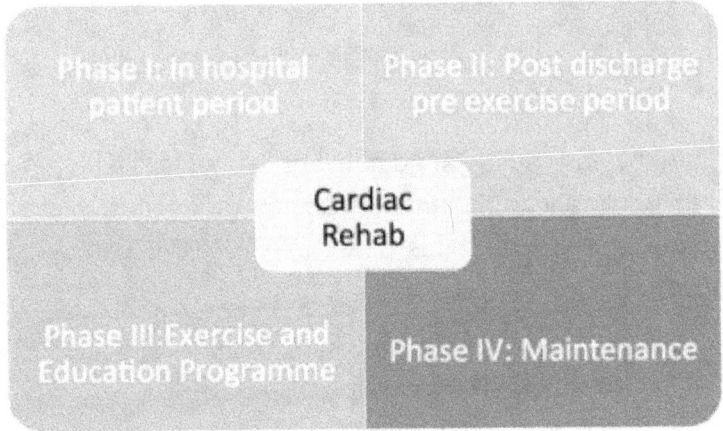

This phase starts while you are still in the hospital. You may:

- Start by walking in your room and then in the hall.
- Do some simple exercises with a therapist.

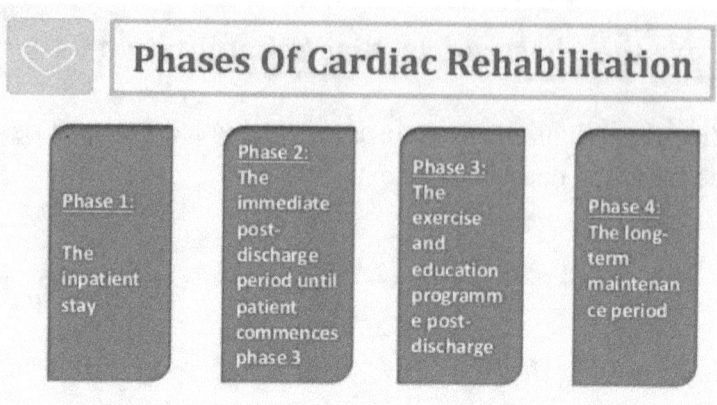

**Phases Of Cardiac Rehabilitation**

Phase 1:

The inpatient stay

Phase 2:
The immediate post-discharge period until patient commences phase 3

Phase 3:
The exercise and education programme post-discharge

Phase 4:
The long-term maintenance period

This phase begins when you go home or to another facility. You will travel to a cardiac rehabilitation center or another place where rehabilitation is offered. This phase may last 8–12 weeks. During this phase:

- You will slowly increase your activity level while being closely watched by a nurse or therapist.
- You will have medical tests and exams to monitor your progress.
- Your exercises may include strength or resistance training along with activities that cause your heart to beat faster (*aerobic exercises*), such as walking on a treadmill.
- Your condition will determine how often and how long these sessions last.
- You may learn how to:
- Cook heart-healthy meals.
- Control your blood sugar, if this applies.
- Stop smoking.
- Manage your medicines. You may need help with scheduling or planning how and when to take your

medicines. If you have questions about your medicines, it is very important that you talk with your health care provider.

## Phase 3

This phase continues for the rest of your life. In this phase:

- There will be less supervision.
- You may continue to participate in cardiac rehabilitation activities or become part of a group in your community.
- You may benefit from talking about your experience with other people who are facing similar challenges.

## Phase 4

This phase is the maintenance phase

- Community based- without supervision
- Patient continue to apply what they have learned

# Follow these instructions at home:

- Take over-the-counter and prescription medicines only as told by your health care provider.
- Keep all follow-up visits as told by your health care provider. This is important.

# Get help right away if:

- You have severe chest discomfort, especially if the pain is crushing or pressure-like and spreads to your arms, back, neck, or jaw. **Do not** wait to see if the pain will go away.
- You have weakness or numbness in your face, arms, or legs, especially on one side of the body.
- Your speech is slurred.
- You are confused.

- You have a sudden, severe headache or loss of vision.
- You have shortness of breath.
- You are sweating and have nausea.
- You feel dizzy or faint.
- You are fatigued.

**These symptoms may represent a serious problem that is an emergency. Do not wait to see if the symptoms will go away. Get medical help right away. Call your local emergency services (911 in the U.S.). Do not drive yourself to the hospital.**

## Summary

- Cardiac rehabilitation is a treatment program that helps improve the health and well-being of people who have heart problems.
- A cardiac rehabilitation program is often divided into phases. You advance from one phase to the next.
- The cardiac rehabilitation team works with you to make a plan based on your health and goals.
- Cardiac rehabilitation includes exercise training, education, and counseling to help you get stronger and return to an active lifestyle.

This information is not intended to replace advice given to you by your health care provider. Make sure you discuss any questions you have with your health care provider.

Document Revised: 04/08/2020 Document Reviewed: 10/17/2019
Elsevier Patient Education © 2020 Elsevier Inc.

# Ambulatory Cardiac Monitoring

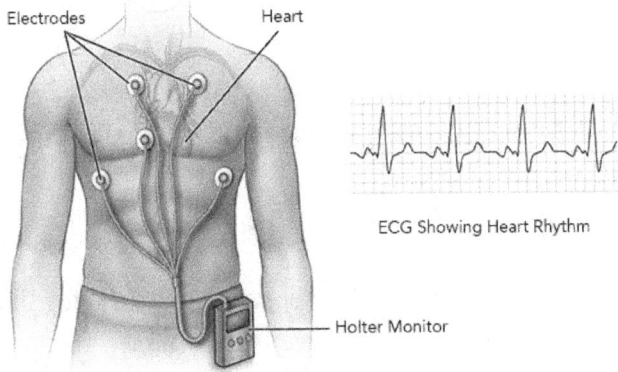

ECG Showing Heart Rhythm

An ambulatory cardiac monitor is a small recording device that is used to detect abnormal heart rhythms (*arrhythmias*). Most monitors are connected by wires to flat, sticky disks (*electrodes*) that are then attached to your chest. You may need to wear a monitor if you have had symptoms such as:

- Fast heartbeats (*palpitations*).
- Dizziness.
- Fainting or light-headedness.
- Unexplained weakness.
- Shortness of breath.

There are several types of monitors. Some common monitors include:

- Holter monitor. This records your heart rhythm continuously, usually for 24–48 hours.
- Event (*episodic*) monitor. This monitor has a symptoms button, and when pushed, it will begin recording. You need to activate this monitor to record when you have a heart-related symptom.

- Automatic detection monitor. This monitor will begin recording when it detects an abnormal heartbeat.

## What are the risks?

Generally, these devices are safe to use. However, it is possible that the skin under the electrodes will become irritated.

## How to prepare for monitoring

Your health care provider will prepare your chest for the electrode placement and show you how to use the monitor.

- **Do not** apply lotions to your chest before monitoring.
- Follow directions on how to care for the monitor, and how to return the monitor when the testing period is complete.

## How to use your cardiac monitor

- Follow directions about how long to wear the monitor, and if you can take the monitor off in order to shower or bathe.
- **Do not** let the monitor get wet.
- **Do not** bathe, swim, or use a hot tub while wearing the monitor.
- Keep your skin clean. **Do not** put body lotion or moisturizer on your chest.
- Change the electrodes as told by your health care provider, or any time they stop sticking to your skin. You may need to use medical tape to keep them on.
- Try to put the electrodes in slightly different places on your chest to help prevent skin irritation. Follow directions from your health care provider about where to place the electrodes.

- Make sure the monitor is safely clipped to your clothing or in a location close to your body as recommended by your health care provider.
- If your monitor has a symptoms button, press the button to mark an event as soon as you feel a heart-related symptom, such as:
- Dizziness.
- Weakness.
- Light-headedness.
- Palpitations.
- Thumping or pounding in your chest.
- Shortness of breath.
- Unexplained weakness.
- Keep a diary of your activities, such as walking, doing chores, and taking medicine. It is very important to note what you were doing when you pushed the button to record your symptoms. This will help your health care provider determine what might be contributing to your symptoms.
- Send the recorded information as recommended by your health care provider. It may take some time for your health care provider to process the results.
- Change the batteries as told by your health care provider.
- Keep electronic devices away from your monitor. These include:
- Tablets.
- MP3 players.
- Cell phones.
- While wearing your monitor you should avoid:
- Electric blankets.
- Electric razors.
- Electric toothbrushes.
- Microwave ovens.
- Magnets.
- Metal detectors.

## Get help right away if:

- You have chest pain.
- You have shortness of breath or extreme difficulty breathing.
- You develop a very fast heartbeat that does not get better.
- You develop dizziness that does not go away.
- You faint or constantly feel like you are about to faint.

## Summary

- An ambulatory cardiac monitor is a small recording device that is used to detect abnormal heart rhythms (*arrhythmias*).
- Make sure you understand how to send the information from the monitor to your health care provider.
- It is important to press the button on the monitor when you have any heart-related symptoms.
- Keep a diary of your activities, such as walking, doing chores, and taking medicine. It is very important to note what you were doing when you pushed the button to record your symptoms. This will help your health care provider learn what might be causing your symptoms.

This information is not intended to replace advice given to you by your health care provider. Make sure you discuss any questions you have with your health care provider.

# Atrial Fibrillation

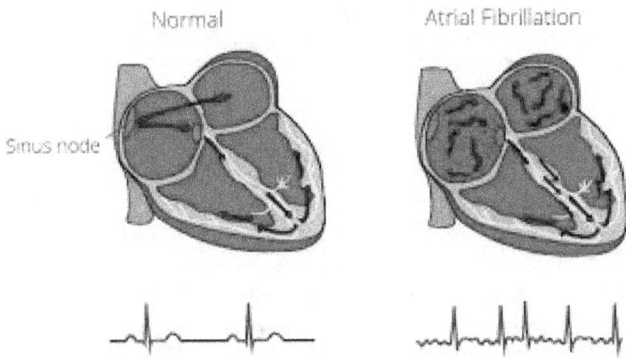

Normal          Atrial Fibrillation

Sinus node

Atrial fibrillation is a type of heartbeat that is irregular or fast. If you have this condition, your heart beats without any order. This makes it hard for your heart to pump blood in a normal way.

Atrial fibrillation may come and go, or it may become a long-lasting problem. If this condition is not treated, it can put you at higher risk for stroke, heart failure, and other heart problems.

## What are the causes?

This condition may be caused by diseases that damage the heart. They include:

- High blood pressure.
- Heart failure.
- Heart valve disease.
- Heart surgery.

Other causes include:

- Diabetes.
- Thyroid disease.
- Being overweight.

- Kidney disease.

Sometimes the cause is not known.

## What increases the risk?

You are more likely to develop this condition if:
- You are older.
- You smoke.
- You exercise often and very hard.
- You have a family history of this condition.
- You are a man.
- You use drugs.
- You drink a lot of alcohol.
- You have lung conditions, such as emphysema, pneumonia, or COPD.
- You have sleep apnea.

## What are the signs or symptoms?

Common symptoms of this condition include:
- A feeling that your heart is beating very fast.
- Chest pain or discomfort.
- Feeling short of breath.
- Suddenly feeling light-headed or weak.
- Getting tired easily during activity.
- Fainting.
- Sweating.

In some cases, there are no symptoms.

## How is this treated?

Treatment for this condition depends on underlying conditions and how you feel when you have atrial fibrillation. They include:

- Medicines to:
- Prevent blood clots.
- Treat heart rate or heart rhythm problems.
- Using devices, such as a pacemaker, to correct heart rhythm problems.
- Doing surgery to remove the part of the heart that sends bad signals.
- Closing an area where clots can form in the heart (*left atrial appendage*).

In some cases, your doctor will treat other underlying conditions.

## Follow these instructions at home:

### Medicines

- Take over-the-counter and prescription medicines only as told by your doctor.
- **Do not** take any new medicines without first talking to your doctor.
- If you are taking blood thinners:
- Talk with your doctor before you take any medicines that have aspirin or NSAIDs, such as ibuprofen, in them.
- Take your medicine exactly as told by your doctor. Take it at the same time each day.
- Avoid activities that could hurt or bruise you. Follow instructions about how to prevent falls.
- Wear a bracelet that says you are taking blood thinners. Or, carry a card that lists what medicines you take.

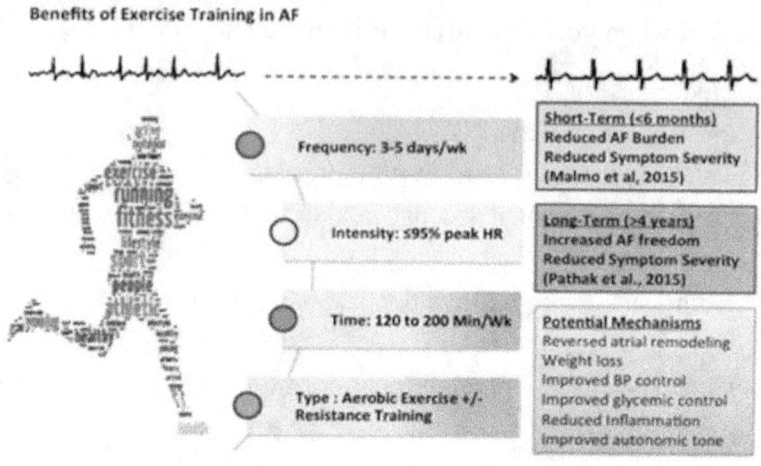

Benefits of Exercise Training in AF

- **Do not** use any products that have nicotine or tobacco in them. These include cigarettes, e-cigarettes, and chewing tobacco. If you need help quitting, ask your doctor.
- Eat heart-healthy foods. Talk with your doctor about the right eating plan for you.
- Exercise regularly as told by your doctor.
- **Do not** drink alcohol.
- Lose weight if you are overweight.
- **Do not** use drugs, including cannabis.

## General instructions

- If you have a condition that causes breathing to stop for a short period of time (*apnea*), treat it as told by your doctor.
- Keep a healthy weight. **Do not** use diet pills unless your doctor says they are safe for you. Diet pills may make heart problems worse.

- Keep all follow-up visits as told by your doctor. This is important.

## Contact a doctor if:

- You notice a change in the speed, rhythm, or strength of your heartbeat.
- You are taking a blood-thinning medicine and you get more bruising.
- You get tired more easily when you move or exercise.
- You have a sudden change in weight.

## Get help right away if:

- You have pain in your chest or your belly (*abdomen*).
- You have trouble breathing.
- You have side effects of blood thinners, such as blood in your vomit, poop (*stool*), or pee (*urine*), or bleeding that cannot stop.
- You have any signs of a stroke. **"BE FAST"** is an easy way to remember the main warning signs:
  - ➤ **B - Balance.** Signs are dizziness, sudden trouble walking, or loss of balance.
  - ➤ **E - Eyes.** Signs are trouble seeing or a change in how you see.
  - ➤ **F - Face.** Signs are sudden weakness or loss of feeling in the face, or the face or eyelid drooping on one side.
  - ➤ **A - Arms.** Signs are weakness or loss of feeling in an arm. This happens suddenly and usually on one side of the body.
  - ➤ **S - Speech.** Signs are sudden trouble speaking, slurred speech, or trouble understanding what people say.

➤ **T - Time.** Time to call emergency services. Write down what time symptoms started.

- You have other signs of a stroke, such as:

  ➤ A sudden, very bad headache with no known cause.
  ➤ Feeling like you may vomit (*nausea*).
  ➤ Vomiting.
  ➤ A seizure.

**These symptoms may be an emergency. Do not wait to see if the symptoms will go away. Get medical help right away. Call your local emergency services (911 in the U.S.). Do not drive yourself to the hospital.**

## Summary

- Atrial fibrillation is a type of heartbeat that is irregular or fast.
- You are at higher risk of this condition if you smoke, are older, have diabetes, or are overweight.
- Follow your doctor's instructions about medicines, diet, exercise, and follow-up visits.
- Get help right away if you have signs or symptoms of a stroke.
- Get help right away if you cannot catch your breath, or you have chest pain or discomfort.

This information is not intended to replace advice given to you by your health care provider. Make sure you discuss any questions you have with your health care provider

# Atrial Flutter

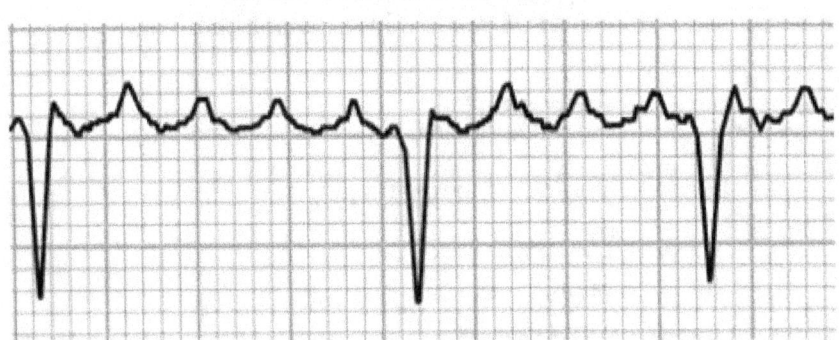

Atrial flutter is a type of abnormal heart rhythm (*arrhythmia*). The heart has an electrical system that tells it how to beat. In atrial flutter, the signals move rapidly in the top chambers of the heart (the *atria*). This makes your heart beat very fast. Atrial flutter can come and go, or it can be permanent.

The goal of treatment is to prevent blood clots from forming, control your heart rate, or restore your heartbeat to a normal rhythm. If this condition is not treated, it can cause serious problems, such as a weakened heart muscle (*cardiomyopathy*) or a stroke.

## What are the causes?

This condition is often caused by conditions that damage the heart's electrical system. These include:

- Heart conditions and heart surgery. These include heart attacks and open-heart surgery.

149

- Lung problems, such as COPD or a blood clot in the lung (*pulmonary embolism*, or PE).
- Poorly controlled high blood pressure (*hypertension*).
- Overactive thyroid (*hyperthyroidism*).
- Diabetes.

In some cases, the cause of this condition is not known.

## What increases the risk?

You are more likely to develop this condition if:

- You are an elderly adult.
- You are a man.
- You are overweight (*obese*).
- You have obstructive sleep apnea.
- You have a family history of atrial flutter.
- You have diabetes.
- You drink a lot of alcohol, especially binge drinking.
- You use drugs, including cannabis.
- You smoke.

## What are the signs or symptoms?

Symptoms of this condition include:

- A feeling that your heart is pounding or racing (*palpitations*).
- Shortness of breath.
- Chest pain.
- Feeling dizzy or light-headed.
- Fainting.
- Low blood pressure (*hypotension*).
- Fatigue.
- Tiring easily during exercise or activity.

In some cases, there are no symptoms.

## How is this diagnosed?

This condition may be diagnosed with:

- An electrocardiogram (ECG) to check electrical signals of the heart.
- An ambulatory cardiac monitor to record your heart's activity for a few days.
- An echocardiogram to create pictures of your heart.
- A transesophageal echocardiogram (TEE) to create even better pictures of your heart.
- A stress test to check your blood supply while you exercise.
- Imaging tests, such as a CT scan or chest X-ray.
- Blood tests.

## How is this treated?

Treatment depends on underlying conditions and how you feel when you experience atrial flutter. This condition may be treated with:

- Medicines to prevent blood clots or to treat heart rate or heart rhythm problems.
- Electrical cardioversion to reset the heart's rhythm.
- Ablation to remove the heart tissue that sends abnormal signals.
- Left atrial appendage closure to seal the area where blood clots can form.

In some cases, underlying conditions will be treated.

# Follow these instructions at home:

## Medicines

- Take over-the-counter and prescription medicines only as told by your health care provider.
- **Do not** take any new medicines without talking to your health care provider.
- If you are taking blood thinners:

  - ➤ Talk with your health care provider before you take any medicines that contain aspirin or NSAIDs, such as ibuprofen. These medicines increase your risk for dangerous bleeding.
  - ➤ Take your medicine exactly as told, at the same time every day.
  - ➤ Avoid activities that could cause injury or bruising, and follow instructions about how to prevent falls.
  - ➤ Wear a medical alert bracelet or carry a card that lists what medicines you take.

## Lifestyle

- Eat heart-healthy foods. Talk with a dietitian to make an eating plan that is right for you.
- **Do not** use any products that contain nicotine or tobacco, such as cigarettes, e-cigarettes, and chewing tobacco. If you need help quitting, ask your health care provider.
- **Do not** drink alcohol.
- **Do not** use drugs, including cannabis.
- Lose weight if you are overweight or obese.
- Exercise regularly as instructed by your health care provider.

# General instructions

- **Do not** use diet pills unless your health care provider approves. Diet pills may make heart problems worse.
- If you have obstructive sleep apnea, manage your condition as told by your health care provider.
- Keep all follow-up visits as told by your health care provider. This is important.

# Contact a health care provider if you:

- Notice a change in the rate, rhythm, or strength of your heartbeat.
- Are taking a blood thinner and you notice more bruising.
- Have a sudden change in weight.
- Tire more easily when you exercise or do heavy work.

# Get help right away if you have:

- Pain or pressure in your chest.
- Shortness of breath.
- Fainting.
- Increasing sweating with no known cause.
- Side effects of blood thinners, such as blood in your vomit, stool, or urine, or bleeding that cannot stop.
- Any symptoms of a stroke. **"BE FAST"** is an easy way to remember the main warning signs of a stroke:
  - ➢ **B - Balance.** Signs are dizziness, sudden trouble walking, or loss of balance.
  - ➢ **E - Eyes.** Signs are trouble seeing or a sudden change in vision.
  - ➢ **F - Face.** Signs are sudden weakness or numbness of the face, or the face or eyelid drooping on one side.

- ➤ **A - Arms.** Signs are weakness or numbness in an arm. This happens suddenly and usually on one side of the body.
- ➤ **S - Speech.** Signs are sudden trouble speaking, slurred speech, or trouble understanding what people say.
- ➤ **T - Time.** Time to call emergency services. Write down what time symptoms started.

- Other signs of a stroke, such as:

  - ➤ A sudden, severe headache with no known cause.
  - ➤ Nausea or vomiting.
  - ➤ Seizure.

**These symptoms may represent a serious problem that is an emergency. Do not wait to see if the symptoms will go away. Get medical help right away. Call your local emergency services (911 in the U.S.). Do not drive yourself to the hospital.**

## Summary

- Atrial flutter is an abnormal heart rhythm that can give you symptoms of palpitations, shortness of breath, or fatigue.
- Atrial flutter is often treated with medicines to keep your heart in a normal rhythm and to prevent a stroke.
- Get help right away if you cannot catch your breath, or have chest pain or pressure.
- Get help right away if you have signs or symptoms of a stroke.

This information is not intended to replace advice given to you by your health care provider. Make sure you discuss any questions you have with your health care provider.

Document Revised: 06/10/2020 Document Reviewed: 06/10/2020
Elsevier Patient Education © 2020 Elsevier Inc.

# Cardiogenic Shock

Shock is a life-threatening condition. It happens when vital organs in the body do not get the blood, oxygen, and nutrients that they need.

Cardiogenic shock is a type of shock that happens when the heart fails to pump blood effectively throughout the body. The usual cause of this problem is a damaged or weakened heart. Cardiogenic shock is a medical emergency and requires immediate treatment.

## What are the causes?

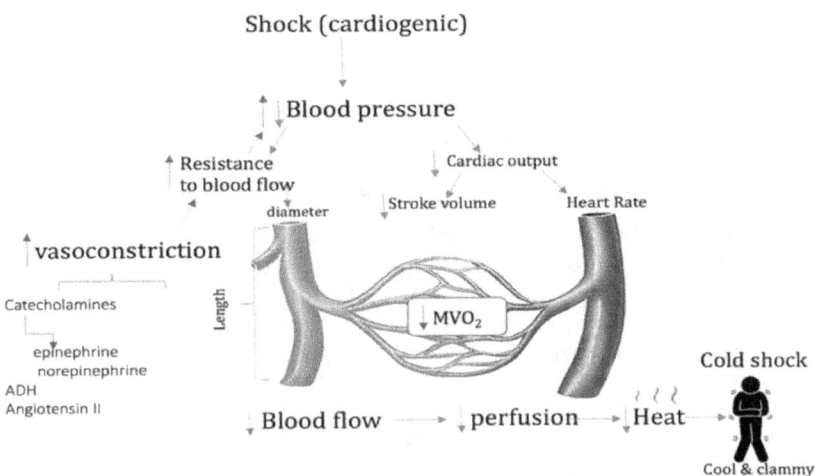

The underlying cause of this condition is heart failure. It may happen suddenly (*acutely*) or gradually if the heart is damaged.

Common causes of acute cardiogenic shock include:

- Heart attack.
- Fluid buildup around the heart that accumulates quickly.
- Traumatic injury to the heart.
- Heart valve problems.

- Certain medicines, including medicines that are poisonous (*toxic*) to the heart.
- A tumor in the heart.
- Infection of the heart muscle.
- A blood clot that has traveled to a lung (*pulmonary embolism*).
- Abnormal heart rhythm.
- Viral infection of the heart.
- Inflammation of the heart muscle.

Heart failure and cardiogenic shock can develop over time in people who have:

- High blood pressure (*hypertension*).
- Diabetes.
- A history of heart attacks or other heart problems.
- Coronary artery disease.
- Exposure to medicines that damage the heart.
- Recurrent pulmonary embolism.
- Genetic defects (*abnormalities*) in the heart muscle.

## What are the signs or symptoms?

Common symptoms of this condition include:

- Low blood pressure (*hypotension*).
- Sweating.
- Urinating less often or a lesser amount than normal.
- Nausea.
- Fainting.
- Weakness.
- Pale skin.
- Cold hands or feet.
- Shallow, quick breathing, or shortness of breath.
- Confusion.

- Weak pulse.

## How is this diagnosed?

This condition may be diagnosed based on:

- A physical exam.
- Your medical history.
- Tests, including:

  - ➤ A check of your blood pressure, pulse, breathing rate, and temperature.
  - ➤ Blood tests.
  - ➤ Chest X-ray.
  - ➤ Electrocardiogram (ECG), which checks the electrical activity of your heart.
  - ➤ Echocardiogram, which uses sound waves to make images of your heart.
  - ➤ Cardiac catheterization, which checks how well your heart is working.
  - ➤ Coronary angiogram, which takes X-ray images of your heart and blood vessels.

## How is this treated?

Cardiogenic shock is a life-threatening condition that requires immediate medical care. Treatment helps to get blood flowing through your body again. Treatment for this condition may include:

- Medicine to make your heart pump better.
- Oxygen.
- Use of a machine to help you breathe.
- Use of a machine to help your heart pump (*intra-aortic balloon pump*). This device is made up of a small, thin tube (*catheter*) with a balloon. One end of the catheter is attached

to a machine and the other is placed into the main artery that leads away from the heart (*aorta*).

- Surgery. Depending on the cause of your shock, this may include:

  - ➢ Coronary artery bypass graft.
  - ➢ Stent placement (*percutaneous coronary intervention*).
  - ➢ Valve repair or replacement.

## Follow these instructions at home:

- Take over-the-counter and prescription medicines only as told by your health care provider.
- Keep all follow-up visits as told by your health care provider. This is important.

## Get help right away if you:

- Feel light-headed or dizzy.
- Have chest pain.
- Pass out.
- Suddenly start to sweat, or your skin gets clammy.
- Feel nauseous or you vomit.
- Have shortness of breath.
- Notice that your skin is pale.

**These symptoms may represent a serious problem that is an emergency. Do not wait to see if the symptoms will go away. Get medical help right away. Call your local emergency services (911 in the U.S.). Do not drive yourself to the hospital.**

## Summary

- Shock is a life-threatening condition. It requires immediate medical care.

- Cardiogenic shock is a type of shock that happens when your heart fails to pump blood effectively throughout your body. The usual cause of this problem is a damaged or weakened heart.
- Getting immediate medical care is important if you have cardiogenic shock. The goal of treatment is to get blood flowing through your body again. It may include medicines, oxygen, and the use of machines to help you breathe and to help your heart pump. Surgery may be needed.

This information is not intended to replace advice given to you by your health care provider. Make sure you discuss any questions you have with your health care provider.

Document Revised: 07/31/2019 Document Reviewed: 07/31/2019
Elsevier Patient Education © 2020 Elsevier Inc.

## CARDIOMYOPATHY

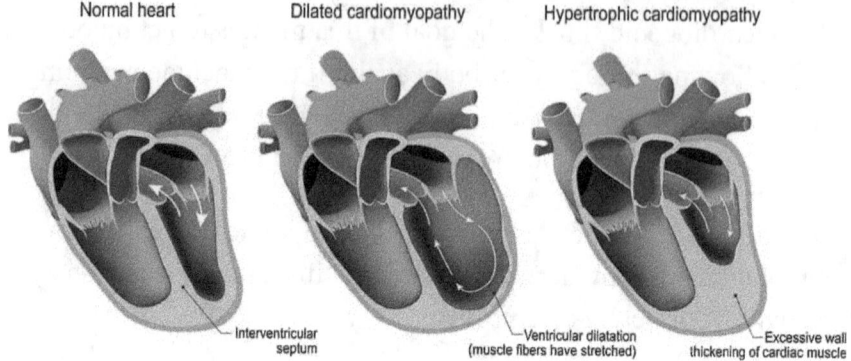

Normal heart   Dilated cardiomyopathy   Hypertrophic cardiomyopathy

Interventricular septum — Ventricular dilatation (muscle fibers have stretched) — Excessive wall thickening of cardiac muscle

Cardiomyopathy is a long-term (*chronic*) disease of the heart muscle. The disease makes the heart muscle thick, weak, or stiff. As a result, the heart works harder to pump blood. Over time, cardiomyopathy can lead to an irregular heartbeat (*arrhythmia*) and heart failure.

There are several types of cardiomyopathy. The kind of cardiomyopathy that you have depends on what part of the heart is affected and how it is affected.

## What are the causes?

This condition may be caused by:

- A medical condition that damages the heart, such as diabetes, high blood pressure, or heart attack.
- Diseases of the immune system, connective tissues, or endocrine system.
- Alcohol abuse.
- Using illegal drugs.

- Taking certain medicines.
- Pregnancy.
- Too much iron in the body (*hemochromatosis*).
- Cancer treatments.
- Protein buildup in the organs (*amyloidosis*), or inflammation in the organs (*sarcoidosis*).

In some cases, the cause is not known.

## What increases the risk?

You are more likely to develop this condition if:

- You have a gene that is passed down (*inherited*) from a family member.
- You are overweight or obese.

## What are the signs or symptoms?

Often, people with this condition have no symptoms. If you do have symptoms, this may include:

- Shortness of breath, especially during activity.
- Fatigue.
- An irregular heartbeat.
- Feeling dizzy or light-headed.
- Fainting.
- Chest pain.
- Coughing.
- Swelling of the lower legs, feet, abdomen, or neck veins.

## How is this diagnosed?

This condition is diagnosed based on:

- Your symptoms and medical history.

- A physical exam.
- Blood tests and imaging studies, such as X-ray, echocardiogram, or MRI.
- Other tests, such as:

  - ➤ An electrocardiogram (ECG).
  - ➤ A portable heart monitor that records your heart's electrical activity (*event monitor*).
  - ➤ A stress test.
  - ➤ Cardiac catheterization and coronary angiogram.
  - ➤ Heart tissue biopsy.

## How is this treated?

Your treatment depends on the type and severity of your symptoms. If you do not have symptoms, you may not need treatment. Treatment may include:

- General healthy lifestyle changes.
- Medicines to:

  - ➤ Treat high blood pressure, abnormal heart rate, or inflammation.
  - ➤ Clear excess fluids from your body.
  - ➤ Prevent blood clots.
  - ➤ Balance minerals (*electrolytes*) in your body and get rid of extra sodium in your body.
  - ➤ Strengthen your heartbeat.

- Surgery to:

  - ➤ Repair a heart defect, remove heart tissue, or destroy tissues in the area of abnormal electrical activity (*ablation*).
  - ➤ Implant a device to treat serious heart rhythm problems or to restore the heart's ability to pump blood.

> Replace your heart with a healthy heart. This is done if all other treatments have failed.

Other treatments may include:

- Cardiac resynchronization therapy (CRT). This restores the heart's normal beating.

## Follow these instructions at home:

### Lifestyle

| Table 1. Treatment options for cardiomyopathies | |
|---|---|
| Approach | Treatment options |
| Non-pharmacological | ● Diet low in salt and fluids<br>● Healthy body mass index<br>● Smoking cessation<br>● Avoidance of alcohol intake<br>● Adherence to vaccination schedules<br>● Exercise training (but moderate-to-high intensity sports should be avoided in RCM and ACM) |
| Pharmacological | ● Diuretics<br>● Beta-blockers<br>● ACEIs<br>● ARBs<br>● Mineralocorticoid antagonists (for example, spironolactone)<br>● Ivabradine<br>● Sacubitril/valsartan |
| Interventional | ● Implantable cardioverter defibrillator<br>● Cardiac resynchronisation therapy<br>● Left ventricular assist device<br>● Cardiac ablation |

ACEI = angiotensin-converting enzyme inhibitors; ACM = arrhythmogenic cardiomyopathy; ARB = angiotensin-2 receptor blockers; RCM = restrictive cardiomyopathy

- Eat a heart-healthy diet that includes plenty of fruits, vegetables, whole grains, and foods that are low in salt (sodium).
- Maintain a healthy weight.
- Stay physically active. Ask your health care provider what activities are safe for you.

- **Do not** use any products that contain nicotine or tobacco, such as cigarettes, e-cigarettes, and chewing tobacco. If you need help quitting, ask your health care provider.
- Try to get at least 7 hours of sleep each night.
- Find healthy ways to manage stress.

### Alcohol use

- **Do not** drink alcohol if:

  ➢ Your health care provider tells you not to drink.
  ➢ You are pregnant, may be pregnant, or are planning to become pregnant.

If you drink alcohol:

- Limit how much you use to:

  ➢ 0–1 drink a day for women.
  ➢ 0–2 drinks a day for men.

- Be aware of how much alcohol is in your drink. In the U.S., one drink equals one 12 oz bottle of beer (355 mL), one 5 oz glass of wine (148 mL), or one 1½ oz glass of hard liquor (44 mL).

## General instructions

- Take over-the-counter and prescription medicines only as told by your health care provider. Some medicines can be dangerous for your heart.
- If you are prescribed a blood thinner, make sure you understand what to do in a bleeding situation.
- Tell all health care providers, including your dentist, that you have cardiomyopathy. Ask your health care provider if you need antibiotics before having dental care or before surgery.

- Ask your health care provider if you should wear a medical identification bracelet. This may be important if you have a pacemaker or a defibrillator.
- Get all needed vaccines. Get a flu shot every year.
- Work closely with your health care provider to manage any chronic conditions.
- If you plan to start a family, talk to a genetic counselor to discuss the risk of having a child with cardiomyopathy.
- Keep all follow-up visits as told by your health care provider. This is important, even if you do not have any symptoms. Your health care provider may need to make sure your condition is not getting worse.

## Contact a health care provider if:

- Your symptoms get worse.
- You have new symptoms.

## Get help right away if you:

- Have severe chest pain.
- Have shortness of breath.
- Cough up a pink, bubbly substance.
- Feel nauseous and you vomit.
- Suddenly become light-headed or dizzy.
- Feel your heart beating very quickly.
- Feel like your heart is skipping beats.

**These symptoms may represent a serious problem that is an emergency. Do not wait to see if the symptoms will go away. Get medical help right away. Call your local emergency services (911 in the U.S.). Do not drive yourself to the hospital.**

# Summary

- Cardiomyopathy is a long-term (*chronic*) disease of the heart muscle.
- Over time, cardiomyopathy can lead to an irregular heartbeat (*arrhythmia*) and heart failure.
- A number of treatments are available for this condition. Your treatment will depend on the type and severity of your symptoms.
- Follow your health care provider's instructions on diet, medicines, physical activity, and when to seek help.

This information is not intended to replace advice given to you by your health care provider. Make sure you discuss any questions you have with your health care provider.

Document Revised: 02/20/2020 Document Reviewed: 02/20/2020
Elsevier Patient Education © 2020 Elsevier Inc.

# Cardiopulmonary Exercise Stress Test

Cardiopulmonary exercise testing (CPET) is a test that checks how the heart and lungs react to exercise. This is called "exercise capacity." During this test, you will walk or run on a treadmill or pedal on a stationary bike. As you walk or run, tests will be done on your heart and lungs. You may have this test to:

- Find out why you are short of breath.
- Check for exercise intolerance.
- See how your lungs work.
- See how your heart works.
- Check whether your heart or lungs are responding to treatments.
- Check if you have a heart or lung problem.
- Check if you are healthy enough to have surgery.

## Tell your doctor about:

- Any allergies you have.
- All medicines you are taking.
- Any problems you or family members have had with anesthetic medicines.
- Any blood disorders you have.
- Any surgeries you have had.
- Any medical conditions you have.
- Whether you are pregnant or may be pregnant.

## What are the risks?

Generally, this is a safe test. However, problems may occur, including:

- Chest pain.
- Shortness of breath.

- Leg pain.
- Irregular heartbeat.

## What happens before the procedure?

- Follow instructions from your doctor about what you cannot eat or drink.
- Ask your doctor about changing or stopping your normal medicines.
- Wear loose, comfortable clothing and shoes.
- If you use an inhaler, bring it with you to the test.

## What happens during the procedure?

## Cardiopulmonary Exercise Testing

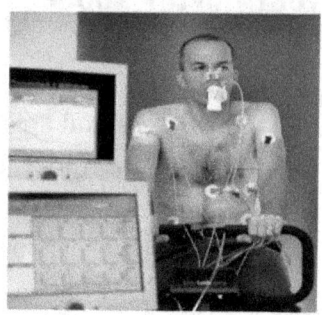

- Standard EKG stress test combined with metabolic gas exchange analysis

- Gold standard for assessments of functional capacity

- Can help determine the cause of dyspnea on exertion: circulatory vs. pulmonary vs. peripheral etiologies

- A blood pressure cuff will be placed on your arm.
- Stick-on patches (*electrodes*) will be placed on your chest. They will be attached to an EKG machine.
- A clip-on monitor that shows the amount of oxygen in your blood will be placed on your finger (*pulse oximeter*).
- A clip will be placed on your nose and a mouthpiece will be placed in your mouth. This may be held in place with a

168

headpiece. You will breathe through the mouthpiece during the test.

- You will be asked to start exercising. You will be closely watched while you exercise.
- The amount of effort for your exercise will be slowly increased.
- During exercise, the test will measure:
  - ➤ Your heart rate.
  - ➤ Your heart rhythm.
  - ➤ Your oxygen blood level.
  - ➤ The amount of oxygen and carbon dioxide that you breathe out.
- The test will end when:
- You have finished the test.
- You have reached your maximum ability to exercise.
- You have chest or leg pain, dizziness, or shortness of breath.

The test may vary among doctors and hospitals.

## What can I expect after the test?

Your blood pressure, heart rate, breathing rate, and blood oxygen level will be monitored until you leave the hospital or clinic.

## Summary

- Cardiopulmonary exercise testing (CPET) is a test that checks how your heart and lungs react to exercise.
- Follow your doctor's instructions about food and drink, and what medicines to change or stop.
- During this test, you will walk or run on a treadmill or pedal on a stationary bike. Tests will be done as you run or walk.

This information is not intended to replace advice given to you by your health care provider. Make sure you discuss any questions you have with your health care provider.

## Cardiopulmonary Exercise Stress Test

Cardiopulmonary exercise testing (CPET) is a test that is used to evaluate how well your heart and lungs are able to respond to exercise. This is called your exercise capacity. During this test, you will walk or run on a treadmill or pedal on a stationary bike while tests are done on your heart and lungs.

This test may be done to check:

- Unexplained shortness of breath.
- Exercise intolerance. This is done for people who have heart failure or coronary artery disease (CAD).
- Lung function. This done for people who have chronic obstructive pulmonary disease (COPD), pulmonary hypertension, or cystic fibrosis.
- Heart function. This is useful for people who have heart disease or heart failure.
- Response to a cardiac or pulmonary rehabilitation program.
- Heart or lung problems.
- Whether you are healthy enough to have surgery.

## Tell a health care provider about:

- Any allergies you have.
- All medicines you are taking, including vitamins, herbs, eye drops, creams, and over-the-counter medicines.

- Any problems you or family members have had with anesthetic medicines.
- Any blood disorders you have.
- Any surgeries you have had.
- Any medical conditions you have.
- Whether you are pregnant or may be pregnant.

## What are the risks?

Generally, this is a safe procedure. However, problems may occur, including:

- Chest pain.
- Shortness of breath.
- Leg pain.
- Irregular heartbeat.

## What happens before the procedure?

- Tell your health care provider about all the medicines you are taking. You may be told to change or stop some of your medicines.
- Follow instructions from your health care provider about eating or drinking restrictions.
- Wear loose, comfortable clothing and shoes.
- If you use an inhaler, bring it with you to the test.

# What happens during the procedure?

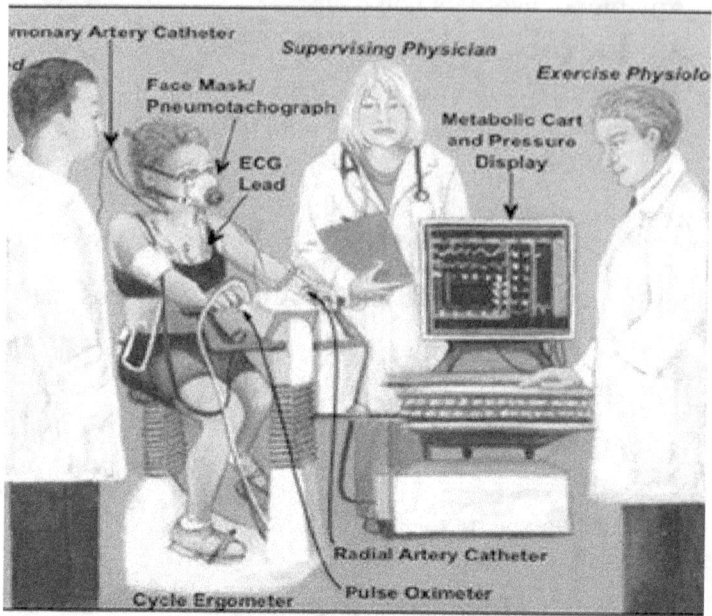

- A blood pressure cuff will be placed on your arm.
- Several stick-on patches (*electrodes*) will be placed on your chest and attached to an electrocardiogram (EKG) machine.
- A clip-on monitor that measures the amount of oxygen in your blood will be placed on your finger (*pulse oximeter*).
- A clip will be placed on your nose and a mouthpiece will be placed in your mouth. This may be held in place with a headpiece. You will breathe through the mouthpiece during the procedure.
- You will be asked to start exercising either on a stationary bicycle or on a treadmill.
- You will be closely supervised during exercise.
- The amount of effort for your exercise will be gradually increased.
- During exercise, the test will measure:

- Your heart rate.
- Your heart rhythm.
- Your blood oxygen level.
- The amount of oxygen and carbon dioxide that you breathe out through your mouthpiece.

- The test will end when:
  - You have finished the test.
  - You have reached your maximum ability to exercise.
  - You have chest or leg pain, dizziness, or shortness of breath.

The procedure may vary among health care providers and hospitals.

## What happens after the procedure?

- Your blood pressure, heart rate, breathing rate, and blood oxygen level will be monitored until you leave the hospital or clinic.

## Summary

- Cardiopulmonary exercise testing (CPET) is a test that measures how well your heart and lungs are able to respond to exercise.
- Follow your health care provider's instructions about food and drink, and what medicines to change or stop.
- During this test, you will walk or run on a treadmill or pedal on a stationary bike while tests are done on your heart and lungs.

This information is not intended to replace advice given to you by your health care provider. Make sure you discuss any questions you have with your health care provider.

# Heart Disease and Sexual Health

Sexual intimacy is an important part of your well-being. After heart surgery or a damaging heart occurrence (*cardiac event*), you may be worried about being sexually active. If you or your partner has any worries or questions about sexual activity, be sure to discuss them with your health care provider. Most people can continue to have an active sex life after heart surgery or a cardiac event.

## When can I resume sexual activity?

How soon it is safe to resume sexual activity—including—depends on the type of heart procedure or cardiac event that you had. For example:

- If you had a heart attack, you may be able to have sex after 2 weeks.
- If you had a complicated cardiac event or heart surgery, you may have to wait up to 8 weeks before resuming sexual activity.
- Ask your health care provider when it is safe for you to resume sexual activity.

## How do I know when I am ready to resume sexual activity?

- How soon you are ready to resume sexual activity depends on:
  - ➢ Your physical comfort.
  - ➢ Your mental readiness.
  - ➢ Your sexual habits.
- Sexual activity involves at least as much energy as climbing two flights of stairs or walking briskly for 20 minutes. It is

okay to have sex if you can do these activities without having any of the following problems:

> Discomfort in your chest, neck, or arm (*angina*).
> Shortness of breath.
> Excessive tiredness.

To check whether you are ready to resume sexual activity, your health care provider may have you take an exercise test. This test involves using a treadmill or stationary bike while your blood pressure, heart rate, and heart rhythm are monitored. The test shows how your heart handles activity.

## What do I need to know about sexual activity after a cardiac event?

### Medicines

- Certain prescription medicines can affect sexual function. They can decrease your desire for sex, decrease vaginal wetness (*vaginal lubrication*), make it hard to get or maintain an erection, or make it impossible to have an orgasm. If you have any of these problems while taking a medicine, **do not** stop taking the medicine. Talk with your health care provider about the problem.
- Talk with your health care provider before taking any herbs, supplements, or vitamins. They can interfere with prescription medicines and your heart function.
- If you are thinking about starting birth control, discuss it with your health care provider first. This is important.
- If you take medicine for sexual dysfunction:
  > Avoid medicine such as nitroglycerin or long-acting nitrate medicine for 24 hours. Taking a medicine for

sexual dysfunction and a nitrate medicine together can cause a serious drop in blood pressure.

## Intimacy

The stress of your surgery or cardiac event can affect intimacy between you and your partner. When you decide to have sex:

- Choose a relaxing atmosphere.
- Feel rested and relaxed.
- Talk openly and honestly with each other.
- Be patient with each other.
- Start slowly, and gradually increase intimacy. You can increase intimacy by doing such things as caressing, touching, and holding each other.

# Follow these instructions at home:

## Lifestyle

- Consider participating in a cardiac rehabilitation program or getting regular exercise. This can benefit your sex life by building strength and endurance.
- Ask your health care provider what exercises are safe for you.
- Eat a healthy diet that includes a lot of fruits and vegetables, less red meat, and fewer high-fat dairy products.

## Sexual activity

- Avoid having sex after a heavy meal.
- Avoid having too much alcohol before sex.
- Ask your partner to take a more active role during sex.
- If you have angina during sex and are not taking a medicine for sexual dysfunction, stop having sex and take nitroglycerin as told by your health care provider. If the

angina goes away, you may resume sexual activity. If your symptoms do not go away within 5–10 minutes, get help right away. This is important.

- If you have angina during sex and take medicine for erectile dysfunction, **do not** take nitroglycerin. You should stop having sex, rest, and wait 10 minutes. If your symptoms do not go away within 5–10 minutes, get help right away.

## Where to find more information

- American Heart Association: www.heart.org

## Contact a health care provider if:

- You are feeling depressed.
- You have pain during sex.
- You are having trouble returning to sexual activity.

## Get help right away if you have:

- Severe chest discomfort, especially if the pain is crushing or pressure-like and spreads to your arms, back, neck, or jaw. **Do not** wait to see if the pain will go away.
- Angina that does not get better with medicine or rest and lasts for longer than 5–10 minutes.
- Shortness of breath.
- You feel dizzy or light-headed during or after sexual activity.

**These symptoms may represent a serious problem that is an emergency. Do not wait to see if the symptoms will go away. Get medical help right away. Call your local emergency services (911 in the U.S.). Do not drive yourself to the hospital.**

## Summary

- Ask your health care provider when it is safe for you to resume sexual activity.
- Consider participating in a cardiac rehabilitation program or getting regular exercise. This can benefit your sex life by building strength and endurance.
- When you decide to have sex, start slowly, and gradually increase intimacy.

This information is not intended to replace advice given to you by your health care provider. Make sure you discuss any questions you have with your health care provider.

# Medical Managements of Atherosclerosis

Atherosclerosis is a disease that results from a buildup of plaque inside your arteries. This plaque is made up of substances such as calcium, fat, and cholesterol and can over time harden, resulting in narrowed arteries. This limits the flow of blood into your body's organs and other various important structures. Long term narrowed arteries increase the chances of heart attack, stroke, and death. This can affect any artery within the body such as arteries in the brain, heart, arms, legs, kidneys, etc. Thus, many other diseases can arise such as ischemic heart disease, coronary heart disease, carotid artery disease, peripheral artery disease, and chronic kidney disease. When it comes to treating atherosclerosis and other heart diseases, the main goal is to slow down the progression and effects of the disease. This can be achieved by various methods and medications. Most commonly, medications such as statins (cholesterol medications), blood thinners, and blood pressure medications are used. Other medications can be added to the treatment regimen depending on the patients' health conditions (Bergheanu et al., 2017).

Statins main goal is to lower your low-density lipoprotein also commonly known as LDL cholesterol. This transpires by its effect on the reduction in intrahepatic cholesterol. These lipoproteins are partly responsible for the buildup of the fatty deposits in arteries which constrict the blood flow. Statins are beneficial for both primary and secondary prevention of coronary heart disease. Current available statins are rosuvastatin, lovastatin, fluvastatin, simvastatin, atorvastatin, and pitvastatin. However, as with all medications, it is important to be aware of the side effects. A common concern with statins is muscle toxicity in which patients may feel soreness, weakness, or tiredness in their muscles. At times this pain can just cause a mild discomfort, but for some, it can be so severe that it affects their daily activities. Hepatic dysfunction has also been seen in small populations usually during the first three months of therapy. Rare cases of severe liver injury do occur; however, this is likely to happen to those with risk factors such as liver disease and alcoholism. Cognitive dysfunction and memory loss have also been reported with the use of statins, but results have been inconclusive (Pinal-Fernandez et al., 2018).

Anticoagulants, also known as blood thinners, such as apixaban, dabigatran, edoxaban, heparin, rivaroxaban, and warfarin are also commonly prescribed. These medications work in several different ways. They prevent clots from forming within the vessels, prevent clots from becoming larger, and often are given to prevent a stroke or a recurrent stroke. It's important to keep in mind that these medications do not dissolve already existing clots. Excessive bleeding and bruising are side effects all patients should be aware of when starting blood thinners. When on warfarin or heparin patients should get their INR (international normalized ratio) test done often to measure how long it takes their blood to clot. Preventative measures such as using a soft toothbrush, using an electric razor, and doing low impact sports are just some ways to avoid excessive bleeding (Harter et al., 2015). Antiplatelet agents and dual antiplatelet therapy (the addition of aspirin) prevent blood clots from forming by preventing blood platelets from sticking to each other. Commonly used agents are aspirin, clopidogrel, dipyridamole, prasugrel, and ticagrelor. These antiplatelet agents help patients with forms of cardiovascular diseases such as unstable angina, ischemic strokes, and previous heart attacks. The medications can also be used preventively when patients have evident plaque buildup. Excessive bleeding, bruising easily, upset stomach, and heavy periods are some of the major side effects. It's key to make sure patients are adherent to taking all doses when it comes to both antiplatelet and anticoagulant medications (Eikelboom et al., 2012).

Lastly, a major marker in assessing risk of cardiovascular diseases is blood pressure. High blood pressure, diabetes, and smoking are all strongly associated with cardiovascular disease. Controlling blood pressure can be done by multiple different mechanisms. Most people will need medication on top of lifestyle changes to keep their blood pressure in control. Multiple medication classes can be used to control blood pressure; these include ACE inhibitors, angiotensin II receptor blockers, beta blockers, calcium channel blockers, and diuretics. ACE inhibitors (angiotensin-converting enzyme) help expand blood vessels and lower resistance by decreasing levels of angiotensin II. This allows the heart to work more efficiently and improves high blood pressure and heart failure. A very common side effect is the ACE cough, where one in ten patients experience a dry cough when taking the medication. Other side effects include increased potassium levels, dizziness, and loss of taste. Examples of ACE inhibitors are captopril, enalapril, quinapril, benazepril, etc. (Peng et al., 2005). Angiotensin II receptor blockers (ARBs) prevent angiotensin II from binding to receptors and keeps the blood pressure from rising. Patients may experience side effects such as headache, fainting, dizziness, and fatigue. ARBs are generally more well tolerated and have less side effects than ACE inhibitors. Some examples of ARBs are losartan, olmesartan, telmisartan, valsartan, irbesartan, etc. (Barreras & Gurk-Turner, 2003).

Beta blockers (acebutolol, atenolol, metoprolol, propranolol, etc.) are used to decrease the hearts force of contraction and heart rate which in turn lowers blood pressure. It can treat cardiac arrythmias, prevent future heart attacks, and treat chest pain. Beta blockers can affect the blood supply to hands and feet which gives a cold sensation. Tiredness, difficulty sleeping, and dizziness are some other side effects (Dézsi & Szentes, 2017). Calcium channel blockers (amlodipine, diltiazem, nifedipine, verapamil, etc.) blocks the movement of calcium into the heart and blood vessels resulting in decreased heart pumping strength and relaxed blood vessels. They're used to treat chest pain, high blood pressure, and some arrhythmias. Common side effects are headache, nausea, low blood pressure, edema, and constipation (Eisenberg et al., 2004). Lastly there are the diuretics (chlorothiazide, amiloride, bumetanide, metolazone, etc.). Diuretics help the body get rid of excess fluids and sodium by urination. This reduces the hearts workload and decreases blood pressure and swelling. Patients may experience dehydration, muscle cramps, dizziness, etc. as side effects. It's important for patients to stay hydrated when on these medications (Shah, 2004).

# References

1. Barreras, A., & Gurk-Turner, C. (2003). Angiotensin Ii Receptor Blockers. *Baylor University Medical Center Proceedings*, *16*(1), 123–126. https://doi.org/10.1080/08998280.2003.11927893

2. Bergheanu, S. C., Bodde, M. C., & Jukema, J. W. (2017). Pathophysiology and treatment of atherosclerosis. *Netherlands Heart Journal*, *25*(4), 231–242. https://doi.org/10.1007/s12471-017-0959-2

3. Dézsi, C. A., & Szentes, V. (2017). The Real Role of β-Blockers in Daily Cardiovascular Therapy. *American Journal of Cardiovascular Drugs*, *17*(5), 361–373. https://doi.org/10.1007/s40256-017-0221-8

4. Eikelboom, J. W., Hirsh, J., Spencer, F. A., Baglin, T. P., & Weitz, J. I. (2012). Antiplatelet Drugs. *Chest*, *141*(2), e89S-e119S. https://doi.org/10.1378/chest.11-2293

5. Eisenberg, M. J., Brox, A., & Bestawros, A. N. (2004). Calcium channel blockers: an update. *The American Journal of Medicine*, *116*(1), 35–43. https://doi.org/10.1016/j.amjmed.2003.08.027

6. Harter, K., Levine, M., & Henderson, S. (2015). Anticoagulation Drug Therapy: A Review. *Western Journal of Emergency Medicine*, *16*(1), 11–17. https://doi.org/10.5811/westjem.2014.12.22933

7. Peng, H., Carretero, O. A., Vuljaj, N., Liao, T. D., Motivala, A., Peterson, E. L., & Rhaleb, N. E. (2005). Angiotensin-Converting Enzyme Inhibitors. *Circulation*, *112*(16), 2436–2445. https://doi.org/10.1161/circulationaha.104.528695

8. Pinal-Fernandez, I., Casal-Dominguez, M., & Mammen, A. L. (2018). Statins: pros and cons. *Medicina Clínica,* *150*(10), 398–402. https://doi.org/10.1016/j.medcli.2017.11.030

9. Shah, S. U. (2004). Use of diuretics in cardiovascular diseases: (1) heart failure. *Postgraduate Medical Journal,* *80*(942), 201–205. https://doi.org/10.1136/pgmj.2003.010835

# Nutritional Managements of Atherosclerosis

In this chapter, will discuss the nutritional non-medical management of heart disease such as atherosclerosis and hypercholesterolemia.

The increase in the level of calcium increases the rate of mortality. Therefore, to reduce the risk of calcification here are the ways to do the nutritional management of heart conditions.

A condition in which the inside layer of arteries called endothelium is destroyed or damaged is called endothelial dysfunction. In this dysfunction, there is inflammation, fibrosis or 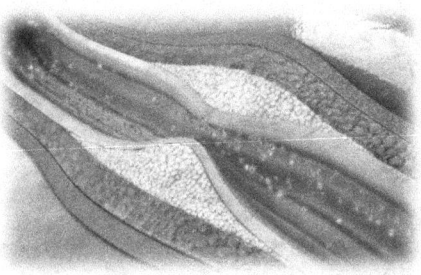 scar tissue formation in the arteries, calcium deposition, plaque formation, or clot in the arteries.

Atherosclerotic plaque is a clot or deposition, which is clogging the arteries. It is composed of 68% fibrous plaque, which is collagen, 8%, is calcium, 1% is foam cells, and these are the immune cells that engulf the debris, 7% are white blood cells they create the inflammatory response, and 16% are lipids. Of these, 16% of lipids 74% is unsaturated fats.

The best test to find out the internal status of arteries is CAC (Coronary Artery Calcification) test or score. It is cheaper and more reliable as compared to the cholesterol test. The purpose of this test is to measure the level of calcium deposition in the arteries, which is one of the best predictors of mortality. Its value should be zero, but sometimes it could be 200, 500, 700 or 1000 or more. If it is high, then specific treatment should be given. For maintenance of healthy arteries, it should be repeated every 7 months.

The treatment protocol to regulate calcium level by diet are:

The first compound is allicin, which is the main nutrient in garlic; it is found that allicin decreases early calcification in animals.

Second is butyrate. Butyrate is a compound that is produced in gut by microbes. Mostly, it is formed by the intake of vegetable fiber but it is actually a type of fat. It is a small chain fatty acid that is produced in gut from microbes from vegetable fiber, and that too, is associated with a decreased risk of artery disease.

Third is lycopene. This is a main nutrient in tomatoes it is a lot in other vegetables and lycopene can decrease the thickness of the wall of arteries and also decrease the stiffness this is why it's mostly said to increase the use of ketchup and it's given to decrease your risk for heart disease because ketchup has lycopene. Now, also if, one had olive oil while cooking. It can greatly increase the amount of lycopene up to eighty two percent, and that is because, like other nutrients, lycopene is a fat-soluble compound that requires bile for absorption and adding more oil to the diet.

Next is omega-3 fatty acids found in fish oils mostly, cod liver oil, which is recommend more than fish oil. It means that omega-3 is good for so many things, but its main action relationship to arteries is to decrease in inflammation. Now the other side, the omega six fatty acids increase stiffness of the arteries and it can increase the clotting factor.

Omega-6 is found in soybean oil, corn oil, canola and cottonseed. The one type of omega six is very friendly to arteries, it does not increase inflammation, and that would be called GLA or gamma lindlenic acid. This is present in Borage seed oil, black currant seed oil, Evening primrose oil so, GLA can help decrease inflammation. It can help decrease thickness in arteries. It can also decrease the plaque formation in arteries.

Decrease the level of omega-6, by avoiding soy oil, corn oil, canola, and cottonseed oil. It can be replaced with omega-3 fatty acids by consuming fatty fish for example salmon, cod liver oil, walnuts a precursor to omega-3 fatty acid and meat.

Another compound is vitamin K2 Most importantly the MK-7, version the consumption of 300 mcg. It's a fat-soluble vitamin, which functions to transport calcium from a place where it's not required like from joints and arteries to a place where it's needed like bones. Consume foods high in vitamin K2. For example natto which is fermented soybean, beef or chicken liver, eggs mostly the yolk, butter, hard or soft cheese. The main purpose of consuming vitamin K2 is to maintain calcium levels in the arteries.

Another important is tocotrienols, which is one form of the vitamin E complex, and it is about fifty times stronger than the tocopherols. The foods rich in tocotrienols are green leafy vegetables. This is very helpful in preventing the scar tissue formation in the arteries and get rid of free radical damage. It can greatly decrease inflammation in arteries and can decrease c reactive protein, which is an inflammatory compound by forty percent and lastly, and most importantly, is doing whatever can be done to decrease and reverse insulin resistance.

The most important factor is insulin level. It is managed by dropping the carbohydrate in diet, which is very therapeutic to arteries. To maintain this the best solution is intermittent fasting or ketogenic diet. High level of insulin can cause inflammation in arteries, which can cause thickness, clot may be formed, or it develops AGEs (Advanced Glycation End products). This situation occurs when proteins becomes unstable inside the arteries. Consuming carbohydrates or omega-6 oil causes this.

Insulin resistance is a condition in which cells cannot absorb minerals anymore. There is a direct relationship between having insulin resistance and having calcification in arteries, and so many of these other remedies are not going to balance until one try keto and intermittent fasting. This is to be done for a period to start making changes but to address insulin resistance, a combination of vitamin K2, tocotrienols, allicin, omega-3 are most important and use the all other compounds as a secondary approach.

Next important factor is to decrease the stiffness, for this increase the intake of potassium. Potassium helps to keep the arteries soft. For this, increase the use of salads. An average American consumes one and half cup of salad, this give 7 or more level of potassium, which helps to maintain blood pressure. A combination of potassium and vitamin D is very effective to maintain blood pressure. Another good remedy for high blood pressure is the use of pomegranate or its seeds in salad.

IP-6 or phytic acid is a great inhibitor of calcification in arteries. It is a chelator as it binds with calcium and other minerals like iron and it helps to pull it out of the arteries.

# Nutritional Deficiencies

Diet effects our body in different ways especially the heart. As heart is the most important muscle of the body that responds to nutrition very quickly.

Heart attack can be caused due to stress. It occurs when the level of adrenaline increases, which leads to the vasodilation of the coronary arteries, which is the main arterial supply to the heart.

Arrhythmias, a heart condition which occurs when there is problem with the pace maker of the heart. It is a neurological mechanism, which keeps the heart in rhythm, and it requires electrolytes. When there is electrolyte imbalance, it disturbs the pacemaker and causes issues like extra beats, missing beats, an irregular rhythm, atrophy or dilation.

Calcium and magnesium work together. The former helps in contraction and later helps in relaxation of the muscles. The excess or deficiency of both of this causes many issues. Calcium deficiency can cause tetany. It feels like a small twitch in muscles of the body. Same like calcium, magnesium deficiency can also cause leg cramps.

An up and down of systolic and diastolic pressure is due to the electrolyte deficiency or it can be a problem with vitamin B1 thiamine. It prevents the heart from enlarging and from different respiratory conditions. The vitamin B2, B3 and B6 deficiency can result in vasoconstriction, which leads to heart attack.

A deficiency of vitamin D3 can also cause a problem as it interferes with calcium absorption. Because it increases the absorption of calcium 20 times in the small intestine. The vitamin K2 and D3 works in combination as K2 helps to control the calcium level in the arteries and the joints. A ratio of 10000 IUs of vitamin D3 and 100 mcg of vitamin K2 taken 4 times a day can prevent the clogging of arteries as both are fat-soluble vitamins and they should be taken with the meal for better absorption.

Another factor is pH; its level can also alter the transportation of minerals. If pH is alkaline, the transport of calcium is not possible. For calcium transportation, an acidic pH is needed.

Nanobacteria are very small microbes in a little calcium shell. It can hide in heart, mouth, and kidney. They are found plaguing in the arteries. A good chelator like EDTA is used to bind and absorb the calcium. It is an option for stroke and other cardiovascular conditions. In case, if the calcium shell is dissolved to kill the Nanobacteria. The use of oregano oil, clove should be used because these are natural edible antibiotics.

The sodium level plays an important role in maintaining the blood pressure. If its level is low, it causes weakness. If it is high, it can increase blood pressure. If there is more intake of refined food, it increases sodium and decreases potassium in turn it will clog the arteries and result in swelling or edema.

By the deficiency or low intake of vitamin E, it can cause the cramping of the heart muscle. This helps to maintain the oxygen level high in the arteries. Therefore, to prevent this consumption of vitamin E rich food such as nuts, seeds, and vegetables should be preferred.

If the consumption of sugar is more, it will result in the increase in the insulin level. By that, the body will start absorbing glucose instead of vitamin C. Vitamin C, which is an antioxidant its deficiency can causes oxidation damage to the artery wall, which can result in the clogging or plaque formation.

## Cholesterol: LDL (Low Density Lipoprotein)

LDL is not a cholesterol. Because fat is insoluble so it needs to be transported for this purpose it LDL is used. It is used as a source to transport cholesterol from the liver to vascular system and then to the cells. HDL or High Density Lipoprotein is going from the vascular system back to the liver to be eliminated from the body.

The body is making 3000 mg of cholesterol every day, which is equal to cholesterol in 14 eggs, or a pound of butter. It is providing raw material for cell membranes whose composition is almost half of cholesterol. As we have a 100 trillion cells in our body. Therefore, it has highly demanded to have enough cholesterol. It works as anti-oxidant, which prevents free radical damage, anti- inflammatory, helps in making vitamin D, and bile salts, cortisol and other sex hormones.

It is also working against infections. It binds and inactivates bacterial toxins. It also prevents the damage from microbes, and works as a band-aid; if there is any lesion in the cell membrane cholesterol will go and fix it.

There are two types of LDL: type A pattern and type B pattern. The type A is large buoyant. So It cannot go in the epithelial membrane and do not cause any clogging in arteries. It lasts 2 days in the body. In this type, triglycerides are low and HDL is high. It is mostly present in saturated fat. Type B is small and dense; it can go inside the membranes and cause plaque formation. It lasts 5 days in the body. In this type,

191

triglycerides are high and HDL is low. It is mostly present in the carbohydrates and sugar.

In type B pattern, it is mostly due to the intake of high sugar and refined carbohydrates. Because of this, diabetics have inflammatory problems, vision issues, and heart diseases. In this type, there is low thyroid, high cortisol, another source is vegetable like soy oil, corn oil, canola, and trans fats, low vitamin C; causes bleeding gums and bleeding arteries, Glycation, it is basically a compound formed by the combination of sugar with proteins or fat which is very sticky and results in high type B LDL. In surgery or trauma, LDL type B pattern is increased, as it is a healer.

## Cholesterol Deficiency

Where the high cholesterol causes many health issues from clogging arteries to heart attack. There is only 0.1% chance of getting heart issues. Low cholesterol is also a more risky finding. It causes depression leading to suicide, cancer, stroke, aortic dissection, short-term memory loss in elderly, susceptible to infection especially MERSA, increased risk for AIDS and for asthma or allergy.

The foods rich in cholesterol are brain, which is a rich source; human brain is 20% cholesterol so it requires cholesterol. Liver and kidney meat, caviar, cod liver oil, egg yolk, butter, and cold water fish all of these are the main nutrients to feed the body and keep it healthy.

The majority of people are vitamin D deficient in this modern era. The root cause behind getting enough vitamin D is having enough cholesterol. It is nearly impossible to get sufficient vitamin D from diet. As only very few things are having vitamin D like salmon fish, egg yolk, mushroom which is only a precursor for this vitamin. The main source to get it is from sun exposure. The mechanism for this is as sunlight is having ultraviolet rays that goes through a series of mechanisms to get vitamin D of which cholesterol is the main part.

Vitamin D deficiency can cause inflammation, high blood pressure, poor immune system, backache, high risk of autoimmune system. Naturally our body mainly liver is making 3000 mg of cholesterol daily. To make vitamin D, but also other important things of not only the body like bile salts; which is stored in the gall bladder with a purpose of helping in extraction of omega-3 fatty acids from the food taken, regulation of microbions, it is in the phase 3 detox in the liver. In phase 3, the bio consumer's helps to complete eliminate it from the body. The main role of bile salts is in prevention of liver cirrhosis and fatty liver. Cholesterol is required as a precursor for sex hormones like testosterone, estrogen, progesterone and cortisol; a stress controller, or anti-inflammatory for the body. The cell membranes of the body needs cholesterol.

Cholesterol is regulated by negative loop mechanism like if intake of cholesterol is more, the production is less. If intake is less, the production is more. Low fat diet is not preferred as it leads to less bile, less vitamin D, and less cell membranes.

www.ingramcontent.com/pod-product-compliance
Lightning Source LLC
Chambersburg PA
CBHW070542220526
45467CB00003B/1030